RC 4
Stua
Para

WN

D0059998

Paradigms Lost

Paradigms Lost

Fighting Stigma and the Lessons Learned

Heather Stuart, MA, PhD

Department of Community Health and Epidemiology
Bell Canada Chair in Mental Health and Anti-stigma Research
Queen's University, Kingston
Ontario, Canada

**Julio Arboleda-Flórez, MD, LMCC,
D PSYCH, DLF, FRCPC, DABFP, PhD, DLFAPA,
FCPA, FACFP, FABFE, FRSM**

Departments of Psychiatry and
Community Health Sciences and Epidemiology
Queen's University, Kingston
Ontario, Canada

Norman Sartorius, MD, MA, DPM, PhD, FRCPsych

President Association for the
Improvement of Mental Health Programmes
Geneva, Switzerland

OXFORD
UNIVERSITY PRESS

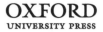

OXFORD
UNIVERSITY PRESS

Oxford University Press, Inc., publishes works that further
Oxford University's objective of excellence
in research, scholarship, and education.

Oxford   New York
Auckland   Cape Town   Dar es Salaam   Hong Kong   Karachi
Kuala Lumpur   Madrid   Melbourne   Mexico City   Nairobi
New Delhi   Shanghai   Taipei   Toronto

With offices in
Argentina   Austria   Brazil   Chile   Czech Republic   France   Greece
Guatemala   Hungary   Italy   Japan   Poland   Portugal   Singapore
South Korea   Switzerland   Thailand   Turkey   Ukraine   Vietnam

Copyright © 2012 by Oxford University Press, Inc.

Published by Oxford University Press, Inc.
198 Madison Avenue, New York, New York 10016
www.oup.com

Oxford is a registered trademark of Oxford University Press

All rights reserved. No part of this publication may be reproduced,
stored in a retrieval system, or transmitted, in any form or by any means,
electronic, mechanical, photocopying, recording, or otherwise,
without the prior permission of Oxford University Press.

Library of Congress Cataloging-in-Publication Data

Stuart, Heather L.
Paradigms lost : fighting stigma and the lessons learned / Heather Stuart, Julio Arboleda-Flórez,
Norman Sartorius.
p. ; cm.
Includes bibliographical references and index.
ISBN 978-0-19-979763-9 (hardcover : alk. paper)
I. Arboleda-Flórez, J. (Julio), 1939-   II. Sartorius, N.   III. Title.
[DNLM: 1. Attitude of Health Personnel.   2. Mental Disorders—psychology.   3. Mentally Ill
Persons—psychology.   4. Prejudice.   5. Social Change.   6. Social Stigma. WM 140]
362.196'89—dc23
2011051889

1 3 5 7 9 8 6 4 2
Printed in the United States of America
on acid-free paper

PREFACE

We have written this book based on our experiences working with the World Psychiatric Association's *Open the Doors Global Program to Fight Stigma Because of Schizophrenia* as well as with other groups worldwide that are dedicated to eliminating the stigma attached to mental illnesses. The *Open the Doors* program has provided a unique test site, involving over twenty countries, both developed and developing. We have learned that much can be accomplished by smaller scale, local programs that focus on the needs and priorities of people who experience the stigma attached to mental illnesses.

We have identified paradigms that have been eroded over time, and that we believe need to be replaced. Our experiences have shown that the stigma attached to mental illnesses is both pervasive and resistant to change. To be successful in the fight against stigma, we will need to adopt approaches that are based on the best available evidence, rather than approaches that have outlived their usefulness or may never have been useful in the first place.

In an area where the evidence base to support programming is thin, research itself having been subjected to the effects of stigma, we have emphasized the importance of critical reflection and knowledge creation. For best practices in the field of stigma reduction to emerge, we must be prepared to abandon familiar but ineffective approaches—those that target stigma at the periphery—in favor of programs that have the goal of eliminating the social inequities that people with a mental illness and their family members regularly face. As in fighting social discrimination, we must consider that this will be a transgenerational effort, and we must plan for such sustainability.

This book is written in two parts. The first part is drawn from the academic literature. Chapters address specific paradigms that we believe require critical reflection and revision. The second part is pragmatic. It draws on our personal experiences in setting up anti-stigma programs and offers a training manual that can be used to guide the development of small, locally based anti-stigma programs that typically have a limited budget. This guide has been used in training courses concerning programs against stigma, successfully used in their development and improved on the basis of feedback from its users, whom we thank for their input.

CONTENTS

PART I Eroding Paradigms

1. Introduction—The Nature and Nurture of Stigma 3
   The Origins and Meaning of Stigma 3
   Consequences of Stigma for People with a Mental Illness 8
   Consequences for Family Members 11
   Consequences of Stigma for Mental Health Systems and Societies 12
   Anti-Stigma Initiatives Are Growing 16

2. Paradigm 1: Developed Countries Have Eradicated Stigma Related
      Discrimination 20
   Mental Health Development 20
   Employment Inequity 22
   NIMBYism, Homelessness, and the Inverse Care Law 24
   Media Depictions and Public Tolerance 28

3. Paradigm 2: There Is Little Stigmatization in Developing Countries 31
   Exploding the Myth 31
   Stigma in Other Cultures 33
        Islamic Cultures 33
        Chinese Culture 35
        Indian Culture 38

4. Paradigm 3: Stigma Reduction Requires Well-Developed Plans 41
   A Case for Enlightened Opportunism 41
   Networks of Practice 44
   Network Governance and Leadership 45
   General Principles, Rather than Specific Plans, Guide Anti-Stigma
      Activities 47

5. Paradigm 4: Science Is the Best Guide for Programmes 50
   Evidence-Based Advocacy 50
   Evidence is In the Eye of the Beholder 51

To Be Successful, Programs Must Target Local Needs 52
To Be Successful, Programs Must Build Better Practices 53

6. **Paradigm 5: Psychiatrists Should Lead Antistigma Programmes 57**
   Mental Health Professionals Are Worthy Targets of Anti-Stigma
      Programs 57
   Stigma in General Health-Care Settings 60
   Mental Health Systems as Agents of Social Control 61
   What Can Mental Health Professionals Do Differently? 63

7. **Paradigm 6: Improved Knowledge About Mental Illness
   Will Eradicate Stigma 67**
   The Nature of Prejudice 67
   Can Prejudice Respond to Nuggets of Knowledge? 70
   What About Mental Health Literacy? 73
   Anti-Stigma Programs as Purveyors of Medical Knowledge 76

8. **Paradigm 7: Attitude Change Is the Yardstick of Success 78**
   The Knowledge-Attitude-Behavior Continuum 78
   What We Don't Know About Prejudice Reduction 79
   How Much Change Is Change? 81
   When Are Anti-Stigma Programs Successful? 83
   Environments Are Not Just Containers 84

9. **Paradigm 8: Community Care Is Destigmatizing 86**
   Stigma as a Consequence of Institutionalization 86
   Stigma as a Consequence of Community Care 91
   Stigma as a Social Barrier to Recovery 94

10. **Paradigm 9: Anti-Stigma Campaigns Work 96**
    The Cause De Jour 96
    Can Social Inclusion Be Sold Like Soap? 99

11. **Paradigm 10: Mental Illnesses Are Like Any Other Illnesses 103**
    Forced Confinement and Treatment 103
    Anti-Psychiatry Sentiments 105
    Violence and Unpredictability 108
    An Illness Like Any Other? 109

12. **Paradigm 11: Stigma Can't Be Beaten 112**
    The Importance of Fighting Back 112
    Overcoming NIMBYism—the "Not In My Back Yard" Syndrome 113

Changing the Way Emergency Departments Do Business 114
Connecting with Teachers and Students 115
Engaging the Police 118
Engaging the Media 120
Can Community Projects Make a Population Difference? 122

13. Summary of Part I 125
Implications for Anti-Stigma Programming—Paradigms Lost 129

PART II Building Programs Against Stigma and Its Consequences

14. Getting Going 135
Introduction 135
Developing a Program Committee 135
Creating an Advisory Committee 137
Setting Clear Goals 138
Creating Interest 139
Acquiring and Monitoring Resources 140
Writing a Successful Funding Application 141
Chapter Summary and Chapter Checklist 143

15. Identifying Program Priorities 144
Identifying Program Priorities Through Qualitative Investigation 144
Focus Groups 145
Steps in Conducting a Focus Group 145
Troubleshooting in Focus Groups 147
Analysis of Focus Group Data 149
Identifying Program Priorities Using Semi-Structured Interviews 150
Identifying Program Priorities Using Surveys 150
Chapter Summary and Chapter Checklist 154

16. Program Development 156
Picking Target Groups 156
Journalists 156
Youth 157
Health Professionals 158
Members of Community Neighborhoods 159
Police 159
Policy Makers and Legislators 160
Choosing a Program Approach 160
Creating a Program Logic Model 161

Including People Who Have Experienced a Mental Illness in Program
    Delivery 163
Families 164
Using Media Wisely 165
    Working with External Media Experts 165
    Working with Television 166
    Working with Radio 166
    Working with the Arts 166
Pilot Testing 167
Chapter Summary and Chapter Checklist 168

17. **Program Monitoring and Evaluation 169**
Using Qualitative Data to Monitor Program Implementation 170
Assessing Change 170
    Specification of Program Outcomes 172
    Setting Performance Targets 174
Devising and Implementing a Data Collection Plan 175
    Data Management and Analysis 175
Identifying Lessons Learned 176
Ethical Issues in Evaluation 178
    Erroneous Results 178
    Anonymity and Confidentiality 178
    Withholding an Intervention in Order to Create a Comparison
        Group 179
   Ethics Clearance 179
Communicating Results 180
Chapter Summary and Chapter Checklist 180

Bibliography and Suggested Readings 183
The Nature of Stigma 183
Evaluation Methods 183
Works Cited 183

Appendix: Inventories of Stigma Experiences 199
Personal Experiences with the Stigma of Mental Illness 200
Family Experiences with the Stigma of Mental Illness 211

Index 221

Eroding Paradigms

Part I draws from the scientific literature to address what we know about the nature of stigma attached to mental illnesses, and the implications of this knowledge for anti-stigma programs. Chapter headings identify a paradigm that has been (or should be) eroded. It is meant as a theoretical companion to Part II, which gives more pragmatic guidance as to how to set up an anti-stigma program.

1

Introduction—The Nature and Nurture of Stigma

Once you label me, you negate me.
—SOREN KIERKEGAARD, 1813–1855

THE ORIGINS AND MEANING OF STIGMA

Labeling is central to the process of stigmatization. In modern times, as in ancient times, labeling someone as *mentally ill* immediately marks them as of lesser value, untreatable, and dangerous. In early Greece, the term *stigma* was used to signify a tattoo or mark that may have been used for decorative or religious purposes, or to brand slaves to indicate their ownership, and criminals to indicate their social transgressions. A sharp stick, termed a *stig*, was used for tattooing; hence the origin of the word *stigma* and its subsequent association with a mark or a brand of shame. The Greeks did not brand or stigmatize their mentally ill; but there is evidence that mental illnesses were associated with shame, loss of face, and humiliation—concepts which reverberate today. In the Christian tradition, wounds that were similar to the crucifixion wounds of Jesus were call *stigmata*, indicating blessing and closeness to God (Simon, 1992).

The uniquely pejorative use of the term *stigma* to signify social degradation probably appeared in the late sixteenth or early seventeenth centuries when mental illnesses became linked with sin. The inquisitorial attitude toward witches represented in the *Malleus Maleficarum* epitomized the negative and condemning attitude toward mental illnesses held at that time (Kramer and Sprenger [1486], 1971). *The Witches' Hammer*, as it is known in English, was written by an Inquisitor of the Catholic Church to help magistrates identify witches (mostly women), and it outlined procedures that could be used to convict them. The witch trials discussed in the *Malleus Maleficarum* contain a number of clear clinical earmarks of mental illnesses such as schizophrenia or depression (Anderson, 1970). While the proportion of accused who had a mental illness is unknowable, it is likely that the root of the Christian association between mental illness and sin was created there.

By the early nineteenth century, most physicians would have endorsed the idea that "lunacy" was linked to dysfunction in the brain. As the century unfolded, etiological theories became centered on the idea of a hereditary predisposition, which eventually overshadowed all other causes as the single most significant etiological factor accounting for "madness." Combined with the Darwinian notion that the most recently acquired characteristics of a species were the most likely to lapse, "insanity" became understood as a regression to an earlier, primitive state of mental development. Environmental factors could explain the first appearance of a degenerative taint in a family, but heredity degeneration became the central organizing concept of late nineteenth-century psychiatry. Important thinkers of the day suggested that heredity was the source of nine-tenths of mental diseases and that people who were mentally defective could be identified with morphological stigmata such as pointed ears, stunted growth, and cranial abnormalities. Degeneracy theory was everywhere until the First World War—popular among criminologists and influential in the eugenics movement. It discouraged early physicians from seeking cures, and it made the austere and crowded facilities that were created to house the insane more acceptable. Because mental illnesses were the result of a hereditary taint, their control was not a medical problem. It also meant that mental illnesses were inextricably tied to other forms of degeneration, which conferred a broader stigma of moral incapacity on all of its victims (Shortt, 1986).

The earliest asylums, such as those found in Spain or Egypt, were originally erected to protect people with a mental illness from the population. For example, in Spain, Father Gilbert Jofré was moved to establish the first asylum in Valencia after observing a crowd teasing and making fun of a mentally ill man. Outraged, in his sermon he spoke of the need for an institution for the mentally ill. Ten merchants offered to provide the funding required, and on March 15, 1410, building began for the Hospital of the Lunatics, Insane, and Innocents (Aldana, Miguel, and Moreno, 2010). While these early asylums were protective, over time, as "degeneration" and "lunacy" became synonymous, incarceration, rather than active treatment, was the preferred method of environmental management.

In the history of medicine, few conditions other than mental illnesses have conveyed such an identity to a group. While a person can *contract* pneumonia, *suffer* from cirrhosis of the liver, or *have* a broken leg; one *IS* mentally ill. The mental illness conveys a master status on the individual that interferes with every subsequent aspect of their being in the world. The person is defined by the disorder: conveying, inviting, and reinforcing stigmatized and stereotypical images. Though we would never consider labeling someone with cancer as *canceric*[1], words such as *schizophrenic, anorexic,* or *rapid cycler* easily roll off our tongues (Nunes and Simmie, 2002). There would be an uproar if people with pneumonia were called *pneumonics* and then prevented from obtaining driving licenses because they might cough and lose control of their cars (Sartorius, 2002a). Yet people with a mental illness are routinely prevented from enjoying the rights and freedoms that the rest of us take for granted; not because they are impaired; not because they are incapable; but because they have been singled out for exclusion from normal roles and relationships.

Contemporary notions of stigma are rooted in social and psychological traditions. In the now-classical work *Stigma: Notes on the Management of Spoiled Identity*, Goffman (1963) examined various forms of stigma, but recognized that mental illnesses were amongst the most deeply discrediting of all stigmatized conditions. Goffman outlined the damaging effects of stigma (including devaluation, status loss, and social marginalization), all of which had the capacity to reduce someone from a whole person to one who was irredeemably tainted. Goffman described stigma as a contagion that was also conferred by association on family, friends, mental health providers, and systems of care. In *Asylums*, Goffman (1961) was highly critical of mental hospitals for their anti-therapeutic and stigmatizing effects and, along with contemporaries such as Scheff (1966) and Szasz (1960), he reinforced the concept that the negative and debilitating consequences of mental illnesses were more a result of the way in which psychiatry was organized than of the illnesses themselves. These theorists ushered in a world view that was deeply distrustful of organized psychiatry and mental health systems—a distrust that is apparent today in the anti-psychiatry movement.

From the original focus on stigmatization as a by-product of the social organization of psychiatry and psychiatric services, much of the subsequent research took an individual focus, emphasizing stigma as an attribute of the person, rather than something that was produced by the social group. The emphasis on personal attributes has been highly criticized by advocacy groups

---

[1] There are a few exceptions among chronic condition labels, which we can't explain. People with diabetes are called diabetic and those with asthma, asthmatic.

who wish to shift the focus from the victims of stigma to the oppressive nature of the broader social group.

Recognizing that stigmatization is a social process, which is inextricably tied to the social relations between individuals and groups, Link and Phelan (2001) have reconceptualized stigma as involving several interrelated elements. The first element involves the identification and labeling of difference by the social group. This is followed by cultural beliefs that link the label and the labeled individuals to negative stereotypes. Labeled people are then categorized in a way that creates a clear distinction between *us* and *them*. Once categorized in this way, they experience status loss and discrimination. Finally, and most importantly, stigmatization is seen as entirely contingent on social structures that provide unequal access to social, economic, and political power. Only powerful social groups have the ability to create and maintain discriminatory practices. From this perspective, stigmatization is the result of a complex social process involving multiple and mutually reinforcing elements.

Sartorius and Schulze (2005) have identified vicious cycles of stigmatization that interact to affect the individual who has a mental illness, their family members, and professional caregivers. At the individual level, a mark or characteristic that allows an individual to be identified becomes negatively loaded. Once negatively loaded, anyone displaying this difference will become stigmatized, with the result that they will experience numerous disadvantages, including inequitable access to care, poorer quality of care, frequent setbacks that can damage their self-esteem, and additional stresses that may amplify the mark and make it more likely that the individual will be stigmatized. This has an impact on the family. The family may experience stress (by feeling shame, guilt, and worry), which can reduce their reserves and undermine their ability to provide the social supports necessary for recovery. At the level of the mental health system, the stigmatization of mental health professionals and services means that they are under-funded, making it difficult to provide high-quality, recovery-oriented care. Medications needed for the treatment of mental illnesses are often not available because they are deemed to be "too expensive"—an idea that indicates that people with a mental illness are deemed to be unworthy of this (or perhaps any) expense. These interacting cycles at the individual, family, and system levels perpetuate disability and, in so doing, promote further stigmatization.

The way labels are connected to cultural stereotypes and the content of these has been a major aspect of the psychological study of the stigma process. Psychological theorists have uncovered how cognitive and attributional processes lead to the development and maintenance of negative and erroneous stereotypes, which are the cognitive scaffolding for stigmatized worldviews. Attribution theory describes a linear relationship beginning with a label, which triggers stereotyped attributions. The attribution may then evoke a negative emotional response (prejudice) and a behavioral expression (discrimination), though this process is not always as linear and clear-cut as attribution theory would suggest (Hindshaw and Stier, 2008). Nevertheless, people who hold moral models of mental illness that are based on attributions that people with a mental illness are blameworthy, are likely to be dangerous-ness and unpredictable, or could "snap out of it" if they wanted to, are more likely to respond in angry and punitive ways. Moreover, those who believe that people with a mental illness are likely to be unpredictable and dangerous are more socially intolerant and distancing, and more in favor of coercive leg-islation and treatment practices (Corrigan, Markowitz, Watson, Rowan, and Kubiak, 2003).

Despite different theoretical perspectives and definitions, "stigma" is often used colloquially to refer to the negative and prejudicial attitudes held by members of the public toward people with a mental illness, which has led many advocates to refocus the discourse on the more poignant issue of discrimination. Everett (2004), for example, suggests that the term "stigma" bolsters the view of mental illnesses as occurring to afflicted others, where the term "discrimination" cre-ates a dialogue that is rooted in civil and human rights paradigms and squarely depicts prejudice and discrimination against people with a mental illness as a form of social oppression—a viewpoint that is reflected in the United Nations Convention on the Rights of Persons with Disabilities (United Nations General Assembly, 2006), discussed in more detail later in this chapter.

From this discussion, it is clear that "stigma" and "stigmatization" may be defined narrowly, to reflect an imperfection in an individual that results in social labeling; as a cognitive-emotional process that draws links between ste-reotyped attributions, prejudice, and discrimination; or as a more complex social process that involves numerous interconnected and mutually reinforc-ing parts, all of which work in concert to marginalize and disenfranchise peo-ple with a mental illness. From the perspective of social theory and public health, equating the term "stigma" with negative attitudes is an overly nar-row conceptualization—one that overlooks the importance of ecology and the structural, political, and the power imbalances that are so integral to the stigmatization process. Throughout this book, we adopt the larger and more complex definition, which has, at its basis, the conviction that the mentally ill are of no value to society or to themselves. Not only does this broader defini-tion resonate better with public health and social disability discourse, it better reflects the day-to-day experiences of people who have a mental illness and the challenges they face in fighting to become full and effective members of society.

CONSEQUENCES OF STIGMA FOR PEOPLE WITH A MENTAL ILLNESS

People who experience a mental illness describe stigma as more devastating, disabling, and life-limiting than the illness itself (Schulze and Angermeyer, 2003):

> *I would do anything to have breast cancer over mental illness. I would do anything because I [would] not have to put up with the stigma* (The Standing Committee on Social Affairs, Science and Technology, 2006, p. 2).

> *Stigma was, for me, the most agonizing aspect of my disorder. It cost friendships, career opportunities, and—most importantly—my self-esteem. It wasn't long before I began internalizing the attitudes of others, viewing myself as a lesser person. In fact, this process began the moment I received a diagnosis* (Simmie and Nunes, 2001, p. 308).

As this last quote illustrates, people with a mental illness may internalize the negative attitudes of others. Self-stigma (or internalized stigma) refers to the loss of self that can occur as a result of being stigmatized. Self-stigma occurs when an individual internalizes negative cultural stereotypes and comes to feel that they are of no value to anyone. This leads to treatment avoidance, a reduction in hope, self-esteem, self-efficacy, empowerment, morale, poor recovery, and lowered quality of life. Self-stigma has been associated with increased symptom severity, and diminished social functioning, insight, and poor recovery.

Self-stigma is prominent among people with a mental illness. In a 14-country study of self-stigma, empowerment, and perceived discrimination among 1,340 people with schizophrenia who were members of mental health charity organizations, close to half (41.7%) reported moderate or high levels of self-stigma. Almost 70% reported moderate to high levels of perceived discrimination, and this was significantly associated with higher reported self-stigma. Factors that were found to be associated with lower levels of self-stigma, such as empowerment or self-esteem, may be particularly important targets for anti-stigma programs (Brohan, Elgie, Sartorius, Thornicroft, and GAMIAN-Europe Study Group, 2010).

Despite the importance of self-stigma, and more generally of the perspectives of people with lived experience of a mental illness, the bulk of research has examined publicly held stereotypes (or public stigma). Understanding the experiences of people who have a mental illness and their family members is essential if anti-stigma programs are to be appropriately targeted and if they are to be evaluated by criteria that are meaningful for those who bear the burden of stigma. Unfortunately, the frequency and impact of stigma experienced by people with a mental illness or their family members has not been widely researched, although it is a topic of increasing interest.

In 1999, the National Alliance for the Mentally Ill in the United States funded a survey of stigma experiences in almost 1,400 volunteers, published with the title *Telling Is Risky Business* (Wahl, 1999). This was the first large-scale national attempt to summarize the impact of stigma on people with a mental illness. In this sample, stigma experiences aroused strong emotions, ranging from hurt to anger, which were seldom voiced for fear that they would be ignored or taken as evidence of mental instability. People who had concealed their illness worried that if they responded to hurtful or offensive remarks, others would suspect them. They suppressed their feelings of outrage and suffered them alone. The majority (71%) also reported that they had denied having had a mental illness on written applications for fear that the information would be used against them. Almost a third (31%) reported that they had been turned down for a job that they were qualified to do, once they disclosed their mental illness. Their experiences of stigma had led them to become more socially isolated, as a way of avoiding disclosure, and had lowered their motivation to seek opportunities such as jobs. Others were trapped in unsatisfying situations in order to avoid disclosure; all of which resulted in considerable fear and anxiety that they might be found out. Approximately one in ten respondents said their stigma experiences had made them reluctant to seek professional help, because they did not want to hear that they were lacking in character, were weak-willed, or that they would have to lower their expectations. Parents avoided seeking help for their children because they feared that the blame of labeling a child would put a moral taint on the entire family. The majority (74%) had avoided telling others outside of their immediate family. Implicit in all of these descriptions was the clear message that stigma had become a major barrier to recovery.

In a Canadian study (Stuart, Milev, and Koller, 2005), almost half (44%) of the sample of 70 volunteers from local mental health agencies reported that they had been treated unfairly or that their rights had been denied because of their illness, and 41% reported that they had been teased, bullied, or harassed because of their illness. Almost half (47%) thought that these experiences had affected their recovery, and 60% thought that stigma had affected their self-esteem. Many (41%) reported that their experiences with stigma had affected their ability to make or keep friends, and 57% thought that it had affected their ability to interact with their families. The majority (64%) reported that stigma had interfered with their quality of life, and 61.4% said they tried to avoid stigmatizing situations. When rated on a scale of zero (reflecting no impact) to 10 (reflecting highest possible impact), the highest ratings were given to disruptions in social contacts (average rating of 6) and self-esteem (average rating of 5.5).

In 2009, the International Study of Discrimination and Stigma Outcomes in Mental Health (*INDIGO) Study* reported on the stigma experiences of patients diagnosed with schizophrenia in 27 countries (*N* = 729) (Thornicroft, Brohan, Rose, Sartorius, Leese, and INDIGO Study Group, 2009). Negative discrimination was reported by 47% of the respondents, most often in making or keeping friends (43%). However, 29% had experienced discrimination from family members, 29% from employers in finding or keeping a job, and 27% from intimate partners. Experiences of positive discrimination, where people with a mental illness received better access to services, were rare (reported by fewer than 10%), but occurred among some families or when seeking welfare, disability pensions, housing, or payment for medical treatments. Anticipated discrimination was reported by 64% with respect to applying for work, training, or education, and by 55% of those looking for a close relationship. Almost three-quarters (72%) felt the need to conceal their diagnosis.

None of the studies completed to date have used a nationally representative sample, so it is unclear whether the stigma experiences reported by respondents in these selected samples are representative of all people with a mental illness. Canada's Mental Health Commission's *Opening Minds* anti-stigma and anti-discrimination program has recently commissioned Statistics Canada, Canada's national statistical reporting agency, to address this gap (Mental Health Commission of Canada, 2011). Table 1-1 shows the preliminary data from a representative survey of over 10,000 Canadians. It demonstrates that the areas most frequently cited as being impacted by stigma are family and romantic relationships (reported by almost a third of this sample).

Table 1-1. PREVALENCE OF PERSONAL STIGMA REPORTED BY THE SUB-SAMPLE OF RESPONDENTS (7% OF THE SAMPLE) WHO REPORTED TREATMENT FOR AN EMOTIONAL OR MENTAL HEALTH PROBLEM IN THE YEAR PRIOR TO THE SURVEY

Survey item	Weighted %*
Self-reported impact on**:	
Family relationships	32.0%
Romantic life	30.0%
Work or school life	27.5%
Financial situation	25.0%
Housing situation	18.0%

NOTES: * Results have been weighted to account for the complex sampling design. ** Personal stigma measures the weighted percent of those indicating some impact of stigma on an 11-point scale where 0 = no impact and 1–10 = some impact.

CONSEQUENCES FOR FAMILY MEMBERS

From the early days when mental illnesses were considered indicative of a genetic taint, to the era of psychoanalysis, family members have been blamed for everything from causing mental illnesses through genetic transmission of defects, to parental incompetence, to harboring dangerous criminals in their midst. Goffman (1963) was the first to describe the stigma-by-association that is experienced by family members. He used the term *courtesy stigma* to describe the social blemish that is ascribed to those who associate most closely with an individual who is stigmatized—though there is nothing "courteous" about it![2]

The proportion of people with a mental illness who are living with family members has increased since de-institutionalization, as the family has again become the primary source of care. To avoid stigma-by-association, family members may keep a skeleton in the closet by trying to conceal a relative's illness from their friends and extended family. In a sample of 156 parents and spouses of people who had experienced their first admission to a psychiatric hospital, half reported some degree of concealment. Concealment was higher among relatives of female patients, patients with less severe symptoms, and those who lived apart from the patient (Phelan, Bromet, and Link, 1998).

In a study of 61 family caregivers (Stuart, Milev, and Koller, 2005), the majority (71%) agreed that people think less of someone with a mental illness, and half (53%) thought that people were afraid of someone with a mental illness. Forty-three percent reported that their relative had been stigmatized because of their mental illness, and 20% reported that they, personally, had felt stigmatized. Half (53%) reported that stigma had affected their family's quality of life; 43% reported that stigma had affected their own ability to interact with other relatives; and 28% reported that stigma had affected their family's ability to make or keep friends. In many developing countries, where treatment from traditional healers or the health services does not produce good results, people with a mental illness are hidden in the house, sometimes chained, or ejected from their homes to become vagrants, surviving by begging and living off food found in garbage dumps (see Figure 1.1).

The shame and worry that family members feel creates stress and, in some cases, a sense of burnout that may deplete their social resources. This means that family members will be less able to support their ill relative, and in some extreme cases, family ties may be severed entirely. Reduced social support may exacerbate the symptoms experienced by their mentally ill relative and promote

---

[2] The term "courtesy stigma" referred to courtesy membership in the stigmatized group or clan by individuals who were the "wise normals"—those who, by virtue of their close association with the stigmatized, knew most about them. The courtesy association referred to their acceptance as a member of the stigmatized group.

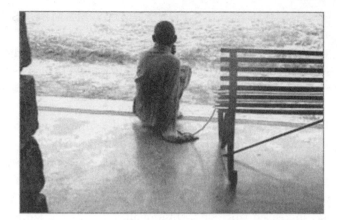

Figure 1.1 Boy chained to a bench in Africa. Photo by Sylveter Kantontaka for the World Health Organization, accessed from http://www.globalmentalhealth.org/gallery.php, November 15, 2011 (Courtesy of Sylvester Katontoka).

a relapse. This is portrayed as a vicious cycle of shame, reduced support, social disadvantage, increased stress, and increased disability (Sartorius and Schulze, 2005).

CONSEQUENCES OF STIGMA FOR MENTAL HEALTH SYSTEMS AND SOCIETIES

In recent years, the public-health importance of neuropsychiatric disorders has been highlighted through a series of large-scale population-based studies. One of the most notable, the Global Burden of Disease Study, estimated that 22% of the total years lived with a disability worldwide were attributable to neuropsychiatric disorders, which accounted for five of the top ten leading causes of disability. Depression was estimated to account for almost 11% of the years lived with a disability, making it the leading source of disability for any single illness category. Anemia, the second leading contender, accounted for 5% (Murray and Lopez, 1996). The World Disability Report (World Health Organization and the World Bank, 2011) estimated that depression was the third leading source of disability worldwide for all age groups combined. Seven of the top 20 causes of disability were attributed to mental and substance use disorders:

1. Hearing Loss
2. Refractive errors
3. Depression
4. Cataracts

5. Unintentional injuries
6. Osteoarthritis
7. Alcohol dependence and problem use
8. Infertility due to unsafe abortion and maternal sepsis
9. Macular degeneration
10. Chronic obstructive pulmonary disease
11. Ischaemic heart disease
12. Bipolar disorder
13. Asthma
14. Schizophrenia
15. Glaucoma
16. Alzheimer and other dementias
17. Panic disorder
18. Cerebrovascular disease
19. Rheumatoid arthritis
20. Drug dependence and problem use

In 1991, the United Nations, through Resolution 46-119, adopted principles for the protection of persons with a mental illness and for the improvement of mental health care, effectively making access to appropriate care a globally recognized human right (United Nations General Assembly, 1991). Mental disorders are the only illness group for which access to treatment is described as a human right. In 2008, the United Nations Convention on the Rights of Persons with Disabilities came into force (United Nations General Assembly, 2006) to promote, protect, and ensure the full and equal enjoyment of human rights and fundamental freedoms for people with disabilities, including people with mental and intellectual disabilities. Signatories agree to adopt appropriate legislative, administrative, and other measures to ensure that the rights of people with disabilities are recognized. The Convention also requires parties to raise awareness about the rights of people with disabilities, foster respect, and combat stereotypes, prejudices, and harmful practices. With respect to health care services, the Convention requires that people with disabilities have access to the same range, quality, and standard of care as provided to non-disabled people.

Despite these obligations, the majority of the world's population still has little or no access to even basic mental health services or treatments. The statistics are appalling. Of the countries that reported to the World Health Organization's Mental Health Atlas Project (2005), fully a third had no specified budget for mental health programs, and one in five spent less than one cent out of every health-care dollar on mental health. Two-thirds of the world's population had access to less than one psychiatric hospital bed per 10,000 residents, and more than half of these beds remained in outmoded custodial institutions. Such

institutions are no longer recommended for the inpatient treatment of mental disorders, as they have been associated with poor psychosocial and clinical
outcomes and, in many parts of the world, have perpetrated egregious human
rights violations (World Health Organization, 2001). Community surveys show
that in developed countries, some 35% to 50% of people with serious mental
illnesses living in the community had not received treatment in the year prior
to the survey. In developing countries, unmet need is as high as 76% to 85%
(The WHO Mental Health Survey Consortium, 2005). Figure 1.2 shows the discrepancies between high- and low-income countries with respect to key aspects
of mental health system delivery. The bars reflect the percentage of low- and
high-income countries that report having specific mental health policies and
treatments.

Inequities in the availability of effective mental health care, and the resulting
high levels of unmet need, reflect a process of structural stigmatization that per-
petuates discriminatory policies, practices, and organizational structures. As
well as denigrating the value of people with a mental disorder, stigma maintains
mental health programs at low levels of priority for governments and funders,
and reduces the availability and quality of care for people with a mental illness
and their family caregivers. For example, the National Institute of Health in the
United States will spend approximately 32 billion dollars on research in 2012.
Despite the fact that some 20-25% of the population will experience a mental illness, the proportion of program funding allocated to mental health and
addictions programs amounts to only 10% (NIH, 2012).

Deterioration in the quality of care for patients makes it difficult to attract
high-quality personnel, which, in turn, contributes to the overall negative

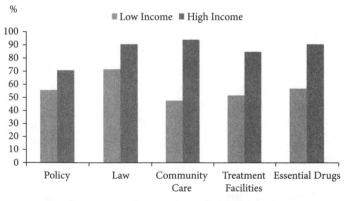

Based on 182 countries reporting to the WHO Atlas Project

Figure 1.2 Discrepancies between high- and low-income countries with respect to key
aspects of mental health system delivery.

perception of services and contributes to treatment delays (Sartorius and Schulze, 2005). In recent years, it has become difficult to recruit medical students to choose a career in psychiatry. Currently only about 3% to 4% of medical students make this choice (Paihez, Bulbena, Coll, Ros, and Balon, 2005). Studies that have been carried out in different parts of the world—such as the United States (Feifel, Moutier, and Swerdlow, 1999), Africa (Dmeteo et al., 2008), and Hong Kong (Pan, Lee, and Lei-Mak, 1990)—all indicate that medical students and young graduates do not consider a career in psychiatry to be particularly desirable. This is a recent phenomenon in the United States, where a larger proportion of students previously chose psychiatry as a career. The reasons for this change are unclear.

There is also considerable suspicion surrounding psychiatric treatments, even among medical colleagues, with the result that they are often portrayed as ineffective or as a form of punishment. For example, a recent news item in the Canadian Medical Association Journal described an ongoing Federal Drug Administration review of electroconvulsive therapy (ECT) devices in order to determine whether they should be banned, subjected to more rigorous safety testing and regulation, or reclassified as into a lower-risk category. The article was accompanied by a colored picture of a man's face from the nose to the forehead, with large white electrode paddles on either temple, with huge, bugging eyes—reminiscent of similar pictures that have been widely distributed by anti-psychiatry groups. A bolded caption appeared under the picture letting readers know that electroconvulsive ("shock") therapy is administered to approximately 15,000 Canadians annually. The article reported that in the United States, The National Alliance on Mental Illness—the largest organization of people who have experienced a mental disorder—testified that ECT equipment should be reclassified from a high-risk to a medium-risk category to ensure that it remains available as a treatment option. They noted that overly burdensome restrictions would make ECT difficult to access for those who need it the most. Also quoted was a psychologist from Texas who testified that it was *unconscionable* to subject people to ECT in the absence of rigorous research demonstrating its safety and effectiveness, calling it a "throwback to the days depicted in the movie *One Flew Over the Cuckoo's Nest*," and indicating that more people are hurt by it than helped (Anonymous, 2011, p. E270).

In 2009, the president of the World Psychiatric Association established a task force to examine available evidence on the stigmatization of psychiatry and psychiatrists and to make recommendations about actions that national psychiatric societies and psychiatrists could undertake. The task force recommended that national organizations should: define best practices in psychiatry and actively pursue their application in mental health systems; work in collaboration with relevant academic institutions to revise the curricula for undergraduate and postgraduate medical training; establish closer collaborative links with other professional societies and with patient and family associations involved in the provision of mental health care and rehabilitation to people with a mental illness; and establish and maintain sound working relationships with the media. The task force also recommended that leaders of psychiatric services and individual psychiatrists must be made aware that their behavior can contribute to the stigmatization of people with a mental illness, psychiatry as a discipline, and to themselves as representatives (Sartorius et al., 2010).

ANTI-STIGMA INITIATIVES ARE GROWING

Anti-stigma programs are growing in popularity, and many countries have now mounted large anti-stigma programs. Some examples include:

• In 1996, the World Psychiatric Association undertook a global program to reduce stigma and discrimination experienced by those with schizophrenia. The program, called *Open the Doors*, had three goals: (1) to increase awareness and knowledge of schizophrenia and treatment options; (2) to improve public attitudes toward those who have or have had schizophrenia, and their families; and (3) to generate action to prevent or eliminate stigma and discrimination against those with schizophrenia, and their families. It was based on grassroots principles that promoted the inclusion of people with a mental illness and their family members in all anti-stigma activities, broad participation from local community agencies, and activities that would be sustainable over time. The program was disseminated in phases so that new centers could learn from the experiences of those going before. Countries participating in the program included Canada, Spain, Austria, Germany, Italy, Greece, the United States, Poland, Japan, Slovakia, Turkey, Brazil, Egypt, Morocco, the United Kingdom, Australia, Chile, India, and Romania. Over 200 different local activities were targeted to well-defined groups, such as schoolchildren, journalists, employers, or police. Targets were chosen based on priorities identified by people who have a mental illness, and their family members, and many have been evaluated for their effectiveness (Sartorius and Schulze, 2005) (see http://www.openthedoors.com).

• In 1997, New Zealand initiated the *Like Minds, Like Mine* national campaign, which combines national media messaging with local-level community action to change discriminatory attitudes and behaviors. There are three levels of outcomes. At the societal level, the desired outcome is a nation that values and includes all people who experience a mental illness. At the organizational level, the goal is for all organizations to have policies and practices to ensure that people with a mental illness do not experience discrimination. Finally, at the individual level, the goal is that people with a mental illness will have the same opportunities to participate in society and in the everyday life of their communities as people without a mental illness. The program provides members of the public with opportunities to have contact and direct interactions with people who have a mental illness, challenges people and organizations to ensure that the civic and human rights of people with a mental illness are upheld and protected, and delivers education and training programs to change discriminatory attitudes and behaviors. The three foci are intended to line up with contact, protest, and educational approaches to stigma reduction. Though activities have drawn on public health and social change theories, those involved consider that they have largely created new ways of doing things and working across sectors and social groups. As knowledge about what is needed and what works has deepened, the focus has changed from raising awareness and promoting attitude change to bringing about changes in behaviors, practices, and policies (Ministry of Health of New Zealand, 2007) (see http://www.likeminds.org.nz).

• In 2002, Scotland's *See Me* campaign was launched in response to long-standing concerns within the mental health community that action was needed to address prejudice and discrimination. In comparison to the *Like Minds, Like Mine* program, the Scots put more emphasis on publicity campaigns to raise public awareness of the impact of stigma on people who have a mental illness and to improve public understanding of mental ill health. Publicity campaigns target the general public and specific groups, such as youth; or environments, such as workplaces. There is also support for local activities that provide materials, advice, and guidance. The model of change underlying the campaign is one that moves from awareness, to attitude change, to behavioral change—a process that is expected to take a generation or more. Though structural and organizational change is not a key feature, as in *Like Minds, Like Mine*, the *See Me* program does work with the media in challenging negative portrayals of people with mental health problems. A communications agency undertakes the creative design work, public relations activities, campaign research, and evaluation activities (see http://www.seemescotland.org.uk).

• In 2006, the Substance Abuse and Mental Health Services Administration (SAMHSA) in partnership with the Ad Council launched a national awareness public service advertising campaign—What a Difference a Friend Makes—designed to decrease the negative attitudes that surround mental illnesses and encourage youth to support their friends who are living with a mental health problem, Public service announcements were distributed to more than 28,000 media outlets nationwide and were aired in advertising time that was donated by the media. Resources that demythologize mental illnesses and videos that model supportive behaviors remain available on the web site (see http://www.whatadifference.samhsa.gov).

• In 2009, England launched the *Time to Change* program—an initiative designed to reduce stigma and discrimination experienced by people with a mental disorder. *Time to Change* is run by three charities with an arms-length academic-evaluation partner from the Institute of Psychiatry at King's College, London. The national campaign uses bursts of mass media advertising and public-relations exercises to convey the messages that mental illnesses are common and people with a mental illness can lead a meaningful life; that mental illnesses are our last taboo and discrimination experienced by people with a mental illness is worse than the illness itself; and that we can all do something to help. In addition to national media bursts, multiple local projects promote mental and physical well-being and raise consciousness concerning the effects of stigma and discrimination. The conceptual framework underlying *Time to Change* describes stigma as consisting of difficulties in knowledge (ignorance and misinformation), prejudicial attitudes, and discriminatory behaviors (Henderson and Thornicroft, 2009) (see http://www.time-to-change.org.uk).

• In 2009, as part of its ten-year mandate, the Mental Health Commission of Canada launched the *Opening Minds* program to change the attitudes and behaviors of Canadians toward people who have a mental illness. The program builds on many of the lessons learned from the World Psychiatric Association's global anti-stigma program. For example, *Opening Minds* takes a targeted approach, focusing on well-defined groups—youth, health care providers, employers, and media. These groups were identified by Canadians with a mental illness as among the most stigmatizing. The program's philosophy is to build on the strengths of existing programs and to contribute to best practices. A key component of the program is to implement and evaluate contact-based education, where target audiences hear stories from and interact with individuals who have personal experience with a mental illness and have recovered or are managing their illness. The goal is to identify effective programs, then replicate them throughout the country. Where gaps exist, *Opening Minds* works with community partners to develop and evaluate new interventions (see http://www.mentalhealthcommission.ca).

In addition to these large national initiatives, smaller anti-stigma programs are also evident in countries such as Austria, Belgium, Croatia, Czech Republic, the Netherlands, Norway, Poland, Portugal, Romania, Slovakia, Slovenia, Sweden, Switzerland, and Turkey (Beldi et al., in press).

Stigma remains a central experience for people who have a mental illness and their family members. Stigma indicates a low value that the social group places on an individual with a mental illness and highlights the broad-reaching consequences for the quality of care provided by mental health systems. However, it is encouraging to see that the awareness of the public health importance of stigma and stigma reduction is increasing, and that anti-stigma programs are gaining in numbers and popularity.

2

Paradigm 1: Developed Countries Have Eradicated Stigma Related Discrimination

MENTAL HEALTH DEVELOPMENT

Most of the industrialized countries, such as Australia and those in North America or Western Europe, have progressed from institutionalized care for people with a mental illness to some form of community-based mental health care, and have done so within similar time frames. By virtue of their greater economic prosperity and progressive human rights legislation, developed countries have many more tools available to them to combat the stigma attached to mental illnesses. For example, they provide significant legal safeguards protecting the civil and constitutional rights of their citizens and guarding against arbitrary detention and involuntary treatment. These protections—termed *first-generation* or *negative* protections (because they preclude interference with protected freedoms)—are reminders of the past, when people with a mental illness were forced into institutions with little protection against abuse or coercive treatments (Arboleda-Flórez, 2008).

The World Health Organization (2001) advocates the treatment of people with a mental illness in psychiatric departments located in general hospitals and the provision of support and services for the mentally ill and their families in the community. It also promotes an increase in the numbers of personnel in mental health care, the formulation of national programs with protected mental health budgets, and mental health surveillance systems. The best of modern mental health systems have reduced mental hospitals in number and size, provide inpatient care in general hospital psychiatric units (with average lengths of stay that may be two to three weeks), and offer a wide array of intensive community supports and services.

The legal rights discourse that marked the institutional era of mental health care focusing on first-generation protections is ill-suited to this new strategy of community care. Modern human rights discourse has provided an important rallying point for the development of second-generation protections that focus on the obligations of governments to eliminate discrimination and social inequities experienced by people with a mental illness. Second-generation reforms mark an important transition from a preoccupation with freedom and autonomy to the protection of citizen entitlements that may be denied to the people with a mental illness who are treated as an underclass within society (Arboleda-Flórez, 2008).

The United Nations Declaration on the Rights of People with a Disability is an example of a second-generation protection. It requires signatories (currently some 150 countries) to take all appropriate measures to eliminate discrimination and promote full and effective participation for people with disabilities, including people with a mental illness. In addition to enacting protective legislation, this includes the abolition of discriminatory laws, regulations, customs, and practices; and the provision of reasonable accommodations and work opportunities for people with mental impairments. The Declaration was written by and with disabled people, and puts the onus on society to facilitate social participation. In so doing, it has significantly shifted disability discourse away from the past focus on individual impairments to a model that views disability as a form of social oppression with broad-reaching implications for justice, housing, education, health, employment, civic participation, and participation in cultural life. Many countries have now enacted legislative protections that are designed to eliminate structural barriers to full participation in social and economic life (Callard et al., 2011).

It is now widely recognized that poverty is one of the major consequences of mental illness–related discrimination (Kelly, 2005), and policy makers in many developed countries are beginning to see employment as a central element, not only to economic security, but to social inclusion. Employment equity legislation in developed countries protects the civil rights of people with disabilities and aims to remove barriers to their economic participation. Such legislation prohibits employers from discriminating against qualified workers in hiring, firing, return to work, and career advancement, and it imposes a specific duty on them to make reasonable accommodation for disabled employees, including modifications to work areas, the use of specialized technology, and alterations of work schedules. Ergo, disability legislation is one important component of the broader human rights framework that is designed to eliminate discrimination against people with a mental illness on any grounds (Callard et al., 2011).

Developed countries have an array of legislative supports available to ensure both first- and second-generation protections and the promotion of full social participation for people with a mental illness. In addition to legislative frameworks, developed countries have an array of community-based programs, anti-stigma initiatives, and monitoring mechanisms to promote social inclusion (Cobigo and Stuart, 2010). Yet, although these tools exist, developed countries have not eradicated systemic discrimination on the grounds of mental illness, and legislation intended to protect the rights of a powerless legion has remained vulnerable to the very prejudices that it is intended to erase (Arboleda-Flórez, 2008).

EMPLOYMENT INEQUITY

Despite employment equity legislation, people who have a mental or physical impairment are more likely to be unemployed, or if employed, they are more likely to earn less than their non-disabled peers. Disabled employees are:

- more likely to be paid by the hour;
- less likely to be a member of a union;
- less likely to receive benefits such as employer-provided health insurance and pension plans; and
- less likely to be in professional, technical, or managerial jobs (Schur, Kruse, Blasi, and Blanck, 2009).

Research shows that up to a third of employees will experience some form of mental impairment during their working lives, most frequently, depression. Three percent will experience a mental illness in any given year, and many more (up to a third) will experience mental health symptoms that may interfere with their social functioning or occupational productivity. In modern work environments, which place a premium on cognitive skills, mental impairments can result in high levels of employment inequity (Stuart, 2007). Large-scale population surveys have consistently shown that the unemployment rate among those with a mental illness is three to five times higher than among those without one. The majority (almost two-thirds) of working-age adults with a mental illness (61%) are outside of the competitive workforce, compared with only 20% of the general population (Cook et al., 2005). The majority of those with a serious mental illness, such as schizophrenia (80% to 90%), are unemployed. If they are hired, they are more likely to be hired for part-time, unskilled positions with high job-turnover and few benefits. Furthermore, any money that they make often jeopardizes their disability benefits, which is an added incentive not to work (Crowther, Marchall, Bond, and Huxley, 2001). A report from the Office of the Deputy Prime Minister in the United Kingdom indicated that psychiatrists are often reluctant to encourage patients to seek work, because, if unsuccessful, they would be unable to reobtain their disability benefits (Office of the Deputy Prime Minister, 2004).

The low employment rate among people with mental illnesses is not due to their reluctance to work. In the United States, 90% of those with a mental illness who were unemployed wanted to work, compared to 76% of those who were unemployed with no illness. Almost half of those with a mental illness (44%) indicated that their last job had ended due to a permanent disability, and 9% were fired. Sixty-four percent indicated they would enjoy a job even if they were not paid (Mohammad, Schur, and Blanck, 2011).

In addition to low employment rates, people with a mental illness who are in the workforce earn significantly less than their non-impaired counterparts. In the United States, for example, Kessler and colleagues (2008) have estimated that people with a serious mental illness (6.5% of the sample) earned approximately half of the annual income of those without a serious mental illness ($22,545 compared to $38,851 respectively). Three-quarters of the average aggregate losses among those with a mental illness were due to lower earnings amongst those who were employed. In this study, "serious mental illness" was defined as: a psychotic illness, a severe depression or anxiety disorder, a 12-month suicide attempt with serious lethality intent, an impulse-control disorder with repeated serious violence, or any other disorder that resulted in 30 or more days in which the respondent could not carry out daily activities in the 12 months preceding the interview.

While employment inequities may be partly due to impairments that limit productivity, there is considerable evidence to suggest that stigma also plays an important role. Employers often express concerns that people with a mental illness will be limited in their ability to perform job tasks, particularly those involving cognitive skills or where the work is stressful. They worry about an individual's ability to interact with other workers in socially appropriate ways, remain reluctant to hire people with a mental illness, and often forcefully challenge (and win) discrimination claims that are made under employment equity legislation (Stuart, 2007).

A psychiatric diagnosis also reduces possibilities for career advancement among the individuals who are employed. Workers who return to work following treatment for a mental illness may come back to highly supervised positions with significantly less authority than when they left. They may become socially marginalized among their work colleagues and bear the brunt of openly negative comments. Colleagues may view the person's workplace accommodations as special treatment or an unfair advantage. To avoid these difficulties, employees who have a mental illness will go to great lengths to ensure that their supervisors and work colleagues never find out that they were ill, thus making them ineligible for any workplace accommodations that could be made under disability legislation. They will find excuses for their absences and avoid employee-assistance programs. Few organizations have corporate policies to effectively deal with mentally ill employees, and few managers have the skills or training necessary to identify and appropriately manage an employee with an emotional or mental health problem. Consequently, the majority of people who have a mental illness who are in the workforce will fail to receive appropriate support (Stuart, 2006b).

The costs of mental health problems in the workplace are only beginning to be quantified, but they are staggering. In 2000, for example, the cost of mental ill health was estimated to be 3% to 4% of the gross domestic product of the 15 states of the European Union (Levi, 2005). Probably a third or more of these costs were directly related to reduced productivity (Liimatainen and Gabriel, 2000). In the United States more workers are absent from work because of mental health problems than because of physical illnesses or injuries. Between 1989 and 1994, disability claims for mental disorders doubled, and they were the fastest-growing area. Approximately a third of the claims and 70% of the total costs were attributable to mental disorders (Dewa, Lesage, Goering, and Caveen, 2004). Loss of productivity at work not only occurs because of absenteeism, but because of diminished productivity while at work—termed *presenteeism*. Depression is among the costliest workplace conditions because it is highly prevalent and because workers with depression usually report for work, though their performance may be reduced. In a study designed to estimate the costs of depression to U.S. employers, Stewart and colleagues (2003) found that over 80% of productivity costs were associated with lost performance while at work.

As these studies show, despite important changes in the legal and regulatory frameworks supporting employment equity in developed countries, people who have a mental illness face significant workplace inequities that have broad economic and social implications.

NIMBYISM, HOMELESSNESS, AND THE INVERSE CARE LAW

A key characteristic of reformed mental health systems is the availability of community-based supports and services. However, the organized resistance to the placement of mental health services and supports in local neighborhoods— the NIMBY (Not In My Backyard) syndrome—has undermined community service development. Local municipalities use zoning bylaws and other restrictive covenants to limit the placement of mental health facilities in residential areas—especially when facilities involve group homes or supported housing. Neighborhood opposition groups have successfully lobbied city councils and local planning groups to limit or prevent the placement of mental health services and supports in their vicinity. Perceived risk of violence from mental health clients and reduced property values from the placement of mental health services in residential areas are the primary concerns. The greater the perceived risk is with respect to these two domains, the greater is the opposition (Takahashi, 1997).

Dear (1992) uses a three-stage model to describe the evolution of NIMBY sentiments. In the first stage, news of the proposal quickly sparks opposition from a small vocal group who reside closest to the proposed facility. In this phase, NIMBY sentiments are expressed in raw, blunt terms, often reflecting an irrational and unthinking response. In the second stage, the battle comes to maturity. Battle lines are solidified, and supporters are assembled. At this stage, the debate moves from private to public complaint, with a corresponding shift in rhetoric from emotional to more objective statements. More measured voices typically express three concerns: perceived threat to property values, to personal security, and to neighborhood amenity, which may include concerns about the physical appearance of people with a mental illness who may be unkempt or engage in loitering, panhandling, or similar behaviors. Residents worry that their enjoyment of the neighborhood will be significantly compromised and that the mentally ill residents will have a bad influence on children and youth. More-sophisticated opponents will express their concerns in terms of the needs of the mentally ill, arguing that the neighborhood is unsuitable or unsafe—thereby expressing NIMBY sentiments under a caring façade. As the opposition matures, victory tends to go to those who are the most persistent, with the period of conflict often lasting a long time. Opponents may apply pressure through neighborhood petitions, letter-writing campaigns, lobbying of elected representatives, media involvement, and formal demonstrations; tactics that are typically coordinated with the public hearings needed to change zoning restrictions. Vigilante tactics that may damage property, or physical assaults on staff or people with a mental illness, may flare up, though they are rare. Usually some type of arbitration process is attempted, using professional and political sources. Both sides may make concessions, or a stalemate may ensue, with the result that the neighborhood wins.

A population survey from Canada (Stuart and Arboleda-Flórez, 2001) showed that fewer than one in ten residents reported that they would be opposed to having a group home for six to eight people with schizophrenia in their neighborhood. The majority (67%) were indifferent, and 25% were in favor. It is likely that the majority who initially expressed indifference could be swayed to oppose community mental health developments by the smaller, vocal minority.

Residents of Long Island, New York, have gained a reputation for expressing some of the most rabid NIMBY sentiments, including petitions to public officials, legal battles, incidents of suspected arson, physical threats, and candle-holding protest vigils. Sixty percent of community-residence proposals made in Long Island between 1987 and 1990 were rejected, compared to 11% to 33% statewide. Half of the court decisions in New York State concerning site selection involve Long Island communities. Long Island also has the dubious distinction of being the only region where a legislative proposal was made (although defeated) to cut funding to all community-residence projects.

In a 1993 report, Arens examined whether the attitudes of Long Island residents had changed once programs were established and communities had an opportunity to learn about the programs and their residents. Residents in the 15 houses closest to community residences were interviewed, and all but four neighbors agreed to participate ($n = 75$). Thirteen percent of the residents (newcomers to the neighborhood) were unaware that a community residence for people with a serious mental illness (mostly schizophrenia) was located nearby. Almost 70% reported that they held positive attitudes toward the home—up from the 22% who held positive attitudes initially—and 80% thought that the residents were good neighbors. Neighbors commented that the community residence was nothing like what they thought it would be, and some had seen residents helping other neighbors. They considered that the residents were quiet, nice, and no bother to anyone. Almost all (97%) reported that they had never had a problem with any of the residents. Most attributed their change in attitudes to having met the residents. The majority of respondents (68%) reported that they would advise a friend to support the development of a community residence in their neighborhood. Virtually all (99%) reported that they had not heard of any problems selling homes because of the community residence.

People often believe they have a legal right to exclude undesirable people from their neighborhoods, and restrictive zoning practices often make this possible. One of the important differences in Long Island was the existence of legislation that defined community residences serving four to 14 persons as "a single-family dwelling," thereby rendering local zoning prohibitions ineffective. More recent fair-housing legislation offers additional protection against discrimination of people with disabilities. Without such legislation, it would have been impossible to place these residences.

A clear and stable hierarchy of preference underlies NIMBY sentiments. At the top of the hierarchy are those who have a physical or sensory impairment, and at the bottom are people with a mental illness and ex-convicts. This hierarchy not only exists among members of the general population, but it has been shown to exist among health and helping professions, as well as among disabled people themselves, all of whom distance themselves from groups lower on the hierarchy. This means that those lowest on the hierarchy are the most vulnerable to the vagaries of social policy and may have little political support from other disabled groups who are also fighting for the elimination of discrimina-tory practices within society (Deal, 2003).

Until the deinstitutionalization era, housing for people with a mental illness was the responsibility of large psychiatric hospitals. Prior to that time, those who were in the community but not living within family units were left unsup-ported. Since the advent of short-stay units in general hospitals and community mental health care, having stable and affordable housing has been recognized as a key to recovery—and a significant policy challenge. Failure to create sta-ble housing alternatives means that a large number of people (it has been esti-mated as up to one-third) must remain in hospitals unnecessarily. Others cycle through emergency rooms and general hospitals in costly and inappropriate stays. Still others have been placed in custodial alternatives to hospitals, such as nursing homes or boarding homes, which lack appropriate rehabilitation or treatment supports (Carling, 1990).

Many people with a mental illness live in unsatisfactory housing that fails to meet minimum standards of quality, and is marginalized to high-crime neighborhoods where they may be victimized or bullied. Many are homeless. Though it is difficult to quantify the number of people who are homeless at any given time, homelessness appears to be on the increase. Leff (2001) reports that the number of homeless people in England doubled during the 1980s to about 400,000. This was partly due to the reduction of low-cost housing, and partly due to the closure of direct-access hostels that had served as the unacknowl-edged asylums for large numbers of people with mental illnesses after hospi-tal closures in the 1950s and 1960s. Canadian statistics tell a similar story. In the 2001 Census, 14,145 people reported that they had used a homeless shelter at some time. In the 2006 Census, this had risen to 19,630—up 39% (Shortt, Hwang, Stuart, Bedore, Zurba, and Darling, 2008). In the United States, Torrey has estimated that 6% of people with schizophrenia are homeless or live in shelters, 6% live in jails or prisons, 5% to 6% live in hospitals, 10% in nursing homes, 25% with a family member, 20% in supervised housing, and 28% liv-ing independently (Torrey, 1995). In a statewide survey of case-managers of 844 people who had been deinstitutionalized in upstate New York, 34% were living in residences that were in below-average physical condition, 23% were in residences that were considered to be poor, and 14% were in housing that was inappropriate to their needs. Poor housing was significantly related to poor community outcomes (Baker and Douglas, 1990) including the transinstitu-tionalization of people with a mental illness into prisons, nursing homes, and other forms of institutional care.

Critics view the inadequate housing for people with a mental illness, par-ticularly those with a serious mental illness, as harsh testimony to a poorly functioning, fragmented, and limited community mental health system (Stuart and Arboleda-Flórez, 2001). Service provision has stalled owing to a lack of policies, weak political will, inadequate funding, unaffordable housing, barriers to accessing social and health services, lack of outreach by community mental health services, and the misguided belief, by some, that homeless people prefer living on the streets to having stable and affordable accommodation. A significant portion of homeless people (one-third to one-half) do not know where to go for mental health services (Stuart and Arboleda-Flórez, 2000), and primary care systems, even in countries such as Canada with universal access to care, are inadequate to meet their needs. This is an example of the *inverse care law*, where the availability of good medical care is inversely related to the needs of the population (Shortt et al., 2008).

MEDIA DEPICTIONS AND PUBLIC TOLERANCE

Virtually everyone in a developed country has routine access to at least one television set. For example, according to statistics compiled by TV-Free America, 99% of American households have at least one television set, with the average household having more than two. The average American spends more than four hours each day watching television. In a 65-year lifespan, that amounts to over nine years of television viewing. This is to say nothing of the 6 million videos that are rented daily. The average American youth spends 1,500 hours each year watching television, compared to 900 hours in school. By the time a child finishes elementary school, they will have witnessed approximately 8,000 television murders; and by the time they are 18, they will have seen approximately 200,000 violent acts. Over half of all broadcast items (54%) are devoted to stories about crime, disaster, and war, whereas less than a percent are public service announcements (Anonymous, 2011).

Stigmatizing portrayals that link violence and criminality to mental illnesses are regular features of prime time television. Stigmatizing portrayals of "odd" behavior also find regular expression in children's television. The news and entertainment media have produced a vast store of negative imagery containing malignant depictions of madness and horrifying misinformation concerning the use of psychiatric treatments. Indeed, the message that mental illness causes violence has been consistent since the early days of television (Stuart, 2006a).

Sensationalized fictional images of mental illness and the mentally ill are highly memorable. Mentally ill characters are portrayed as more violent than other characters and significantly more violent than real people with a mental illness. With this steady diet of information linking mental illness to violence, television portrayals do little to convince the viewing public that someone with a mental illness could recover, could become a productive member of society, or could be someone one would want to interact with in the context of a friendship, romance, or marriage. Television characters who have a mental illness are typically portrayed as being friendless, with no family connections, and completely disenfranchised from social life. In children's television, characters who display odd or unstable behavior are portrayed as objects of amusement, derision, or fear. Disparaging terms are used to link mental illnesses to a loss of control. These broad and ill-defined images—lacking in specific symptoms or diagnoses—invite negative generalizations to all people with a mental illness. Even very young children can express ideas about psychiatry and psychiatrists. When primary-school students in Canada were asked by their teacher to draw a psychiatrist, not only did they know what a psychiatrist was, they captured notions of white coats, brains, and perhaps even brainwashing.

News media are among the most frequently cited sources of health and mental health information. Like their entertainment counterparts, news media also emphasize the violent, delusional, and irrational behavior of people; often linking these qualities to mental illnesses. Many headlines are sensationalized in order to catch attention. However, even well-balanced journalistic accounts can contribute and reinforce negative imagery that has been accrued through other sources. By retelling a single dramatic event multiple times, news media create exaggerated expectations among members of the public that the mentally ill are violent. Finally, the news media introduce bias by limiting perspectives. Rarely will someone with a mental illness, a mental health professional, or a family member be interviewed to provide context or to correct inaccuracies—a practice that would be considered highly unusual—and incomplete—when following any other storyline.

As a result of media imagery, the public fear those with a mental illness and want to maintain a safe social distance. Figure 2.1 shows the percentage of a random sample of Canadians (1,653 respondents from Alberta) who indicated that they would be upset or concerned about interacting with someone who had schizophrenia, in various social relationships. The closer and more intimate the relationship, the higher the expressed level of discomfort and desire for social distance (Stuart and Arboleda-Flórez, 2001).

In summary, even though developed countries have implemented progressive legislative and human rights frameworks that broadly protect the civil rights of people with disabilities, they have not eradicated the stigma related to mental disorders. People with mental illnesses experience a pernicious form

% of 1653 Canadians Expressing Social Distance

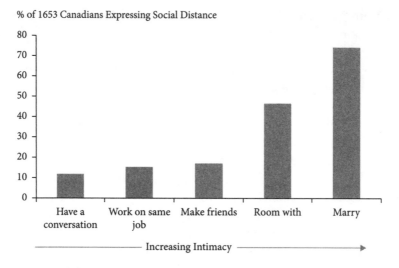

Figure 2.1 Social distance from someone with schizophrenia, expressed by a random sample of 1,653 Canadians.

of discrimination that results in serious inequities in key areas of life, such as employment, housing, and social relationships. In developed countries, the majority of health and mental health information comes from the media, where the mentally ill are regularly depicted as violent and unpredictable, thus reinforcing negative stereotypes that generate fear, intolerance, and social distance.

3

Paradigm 2: There Is Little Stigmatization in Developing Countries

EXPLODING THE MYTH

It is often said that stigma occurs much less frequently in developing countries, where life is considered to be simpler, where strong family values still prevail, and where different religious world views are more accepting of non-medical explanations for mental illnesses. In China, for example, Cheung (1990) attributes this romanticized impression to early reports of the grassroots health-care systems first documented by Western visitors and to later reports by Chinese health officials on model community mental-health-care systems in several large Chinese cities. Leff and Warner (2006) have argued that families in developing countries are more tolerant and accepting toward psychiatric symptoms and impairments caused by schizophrenia. Cooperative family enterprises and agriculture are also more common in developing economies, with the result that people with a mental illness may have more opportunities to contribute to the family income, even when significantly impaired. Finally, in many traditional cultures, mental illnesses are still ascribed to spirits or to a spell (such as the "evil eye") cast upon the person by an enemy or witch, with the result that people who are mentally ill are absolved of blame and criticism and more accepted by their social groups.

In 1967, the World Health Organization initiated a set of studies in schizophrenia. The first of these—the International Pilot Study of Schizophrenia (IPSS) examined three questions: whether schizophrenia could be found in all cultures; whether collaborative studies using standardized instruments were feasible in psychiatry; and whether psychiatrists, despite belonging to different psychiatric schools of thought, could carry out such studies in a reliable manner. The IPSS and the following work on the determinants of outcomes in schizophrenia involved both developed and developing countries. A consistent and provocative finding—documented with increasing precision over the years—was that patients in developing countries had more favorable outcomes than those in

Europe and the United States. After two years of follow-up, over half of the patients living in non-industrialized centers (52%) showed the "best" or most favorable pattern of recovery compared to 39% in industrialized centers. A five-year follow-up found that 73% of patients in developing countries had the "best" pattern of recovery, compared to 52% in developed centers. Similar findings were confirmed in subsequent, more controlled studies (Sartorius, 1996). The robustness with which this finding has emerged and reemerged demonstrates the important role played by culture in influencing the course and outcome of serious mental illnesses, particularly in countries with high family involvement and support (Hopper, Harrison, Janca, and Sartorius, 2007).

However, despite the mentally ill population's opportunities for greater social integration in family and economic life, stigma can still play out in harsh and devastating ways in the developing world. Kadri (2005) conducted a detailed review of stigma studies in various developing societies and found that in all of the cultures represented, stigma was among the main reasons for legislators' refusal to allocate enough funding for appropriate care of mental illnesses, and insurance companies' failure to provide sufficient coverage for the treatment of mental illnesses. The stigma of mental illness made neighbors prevent people with a mental illness from living in their communities, and kept employers from offering people with a mental illness a job. In some countries, families cope by chaining their relative to immovable structures in their backyard or on the street. In other cases, they are caged, beaten, maltreated, or thrown out of their houses to be mauled and eaten by wild animals (Lee, 2002).

Studies conducted in different parts of the world, such as Africa, Latin America, the Caribbean, have shown that people with mental illnesses are not equally valued. Thornicroft and colleagues (2009) have documented the stigma experiences of 732 people who received treatment for schizophrenia, from 27 developing and developed countries. Negative discrimination was experienced by almost half the respondents in making or keeping friends (47%), nearly half from family members (43%), almost a third in finding or keeping a job (29%), and over one-fourth in intimate relationships (27%). Sixty-four percent anticipated that they would be discriminated against in applying for work training or education, and 55% in close relationships. Almost three-quarters (72%) reported that they felt the need to conceal their diagnosis. The effects of discrimination were evident across a broad range of daily experiences with family, friends, and work (for example) in all of the countries studied. An interesting finding was that experienced-discrimination scores varied across countries, but anticipated-discrimination scores did not. A second interesting finding was that over a third of participants *anticipated* discrimination in job-seeking and in developing close personal relationships, but did not report *having* any discrimination experiences in these areas. This may reflect the effects of self-stigma, where individuals internalize cultural stereotypes and come to believe they will be treated unfairly. Instances involving positive discrimination were rare.

STIGMA IN OTHER CULTURES

There are three great traditions in medicine outside of Europe and North America associated with distinct civilizations and religions that provide a different interpretative system for the understanding and management of mental illnesses, leading to different forms of social stigma: Islamic cultures, China, and India (Okasha, Arboleda-Flórez, and Sartorius, 2000).

Islamic Cultures

Historically, Islamic cultures have viewed mental disturbances as illnesses with no particular moral meaning, guilt, or shame attached. The primary responsibility for the care of the mentally ill rested with the family, which appears to have been supportive and tolerant. Confinement of the mentally ill was resisted unless the individual was a serious danger to self or others. Early Islamic hospitals included sections for the mentally ill, which were open to visitors, but unpleasant. Patients—the most seriously disturbed—were held in restraints. The sections had walls that were reinforced with heavy wood and iron, and keepers were equipped with whips, which they used when a patient became agitated or violent. Although folk beliefs and traditions equated madness with evil spirits, mental hospital units were places of confinement where physicians practiced their physiologically oriented medicine with diversions such as dancing, theatrical performances, and recitations. In some hospitals, patients were led to the mosque to pray. So while, patients were restrained and sometimes beaten, the systematic abuses that accompanied the rise of European asylums during the period of the "Great Confinement" in the 17th century were not evident (Dols, 1987), suggesting that mental illnesses did not elicit as much stigma in the Islamic world as in other societies (Fabrega, 1991).

Research on the stigma attributed to mental illnesses in the modern Islamic world is limited. However, despite more tolerant religious and historical traditions, it would appear that in modern Islamic societies, people with mental illnesses, particularly serious illnesses, and their families do suffer considerable stigma. In a study of 100 family members of patients with schizophrenia in Casablanca, Morocco, most family members (87%) reported experiencing stigma because of their relative's illness. This included maltreatment (41%), mockery (29%), and distrust (15%), causing psychological, sleep, and relational disturbances (72%). Only a third of the family members thought that schizo-phrenia had a biological basis, and one in four considered the illness to be caused by sorcery (Kadri, Manoudi, Berrada, and Moussaoui, 2004). Similar results were obtained in Oman (Al-Adawi et al., 2002), where medical students and members of the general public (though not relatives) favored the role of spirits as etiological agents in mental illness. The majority of those sampled thought that people with a mental illness had particular physical characteristics that set them apart from those without a mental illness, and that facilities for psychiatric care should be located far away from communities. These findings suggest a strong undercurrent of social intolerance.

Mental illnesses are not based on modern biological or genetic explanations and are often viewed as the result of supernatural forces. In the Koran, the most common word used to refer to those who are insane is *majnoon*, which is derived from the Arabic word *jinn*, referring to a supernatural spirit. The Islamic concept of the insane is that the individual is possessed by a *jinn*. The *jinn* is a supernatural spirit that has the power of assuming human and animal forms that can be either good or bad (Okasha, 1999). In a qualitative study of Muslim people living in Britain (Weatherhead and Daiches, 2010), religious understandings of the etiology of mental illnesses included punishment from Allah, reactions to life stresses, and supernatural causes, such as being pos-sessed by a *jinn*. Prayer and support of family and friends were highlighted as important methods of managing mental distress. Formal, specialized services would be accessed only as a last resort for the patients who were the most dis-turbed and unable to resolve their problems using traditional supports.

Nowadays, in Islamic cultures, one of the most commonly cited reasons for the under-use of available psychiatric services is fear of stigma. Accessing for-mal, specialized services is associated with shame and embarrassment because it indicates that people with mental illnesses have been unable to obtain resolution of their problems through their faith. For many Muslims, secular views held in European countries and Islamic religious beliefs concerning the etiology and treatment for mental illnesses are mutually exclusive. Seeking help from services is a rejection of Allah's healing powers and is, therefore, socially stigmatized.

Unlike cultures based on individualism (such as North America and in some countries of Western Europe), Islamic cultures are more collectivist, where individuals are defined in relation to others in their social group. This means that Islamic cultures may be more tolerant of mental and psychological dis-turbances as long as they do not result in behaviors that are considered to be shameful and out of control. For example, in a qualitative study conducted in Egypt (Coker, 2005), it was not the mental or behavioral disorder, per se, that elicited stigma, but the interpretation of the illness in terms of its ability to disrupt or contaminate social relations via the powerful influence people have on those around them. In this context, the idea of *magnuun* (or madness) was reserved for the condition in which people fight with others, do not think right, and are extremely unbalanced in their behaviors, emotions, and reactions. A high degree of social distance was expressed for these forms of illness, which were viewed as irrational and incurable. "Ordinary" psychological problems were explained in terms of social causes, were considered to be responsive to social support (rather than specialized psychiatric treatment), and were not associated with high levels of stigma or social intolerance. Psychiatric hospitals were associated with high social stigma and indicative of "madness." Consequently, they were not viewed as places for the treatment of illness, but as places to confine those whom the social group could not tolerate. As places for the hopeless, the socially unfit, and those who were dangerous and out of control, hospitals were themselves stigmatizing as were the asylums in European countries.

Chinese Culture

Confucian ethics provides the moral framework governing interpersonal relationships in Chinese culture. Confucianism expects social relationships to be harmonious. Mental illnesses are considered to be a source of dissonance in an otherwise ideal state of harmony. In Chinese medicine, the focus is on the restoration of balance—between the *yin* and *yang*. Excessive emotions are thought to be unhealthy because they are a threat to social order and social harmony (Ng, 1997).

In Chinese culture, mental illnesses are regarded as a moral transgression against one's ancestors and social norms, or as a consequence of hereditary or ancestral inheritance of misconduct. As a result, both the sufferer and the family members may be socially excluded, such as from marriage. Other explanations include cosmological forces, the wrath of gods and ancestors, possession by spirits, hormones, diet, brain dysfunction, and even political ideology. In many rural areas of China, where mental health knowledge is limited, mental illnesses are regarded as punishment from the supernatural or spiritual world. People holding traditional beliefs support the idea that people with a mental illness should be kept away from local neighborhoods and in hospitals. The strong sense of the family also contributes to social stigma in Chinese culture. Not only is a mental illness a source of great personal embarrassment, it brings enormous shame to the family for past, present, and future generations (Tsang et al., 2007). Suicide and attempted suicide are highly shameful acts. The Confucian idea of *hsiao* embodies the belief that one's body is inherited from one's parents. One must take care of it and return it to the earth whole. Thus, individuals who attempt or commit suicide not only damage their bodies, but commit an act of supreme dishonor to their parents and their families (Tzeng and Lipson, 2004).

In Chinese culture, the main reason for the stigmatization of people with a mental illness is that they tarnish the family honor and the ancestors. There is a strong sense of shame and a desire to conceal the mental illnesses from outsiders. Consequently, denial and somatization are often used to hide mental illnesses and prevent their stigmatization. Traditional remedies are likely to be sought, and people strongly resist seeking specialized psychiatric help. Minor mental illnesses are managed as "physical" problems. More serious illnesses result in hospitalization, but only after a protracted period of seeking out all alterative remedies (Ng, 1997).

Chou and Mak (1998) conducted serial telephone surveys of two representative samples of Hong Kong Chinese in 1994 and 1996. Table 3-1 summarizes some of the key stigma-related findings from these surveys. The first items reflect mental health literacy and concern common stereotypes (such as dangerousness), the nature of mental illness (e.g.: as a non-contagious disease), the prevalence of mental illness, and its treatability. Results showed that the majority of respondents were generally knowledgeable, and small improvements were noted across the two years. The next group of items reflect ideas about community care. Despite being generally knowledgeable, a large proportion of respondents endorsed stigmatizing responses on this dimension. For example, over half considered that mental patients should be kept away from the community, in mental hospitals or distant rehabilitation facilities. Although still high, the proportion of the population expressing stigmatizing recovery ideas improved in the second survey year. The last two items loaded on a separate factor called a *living factor*. These reflected respondents' desire for social distance. Both items were endorsed by a large proportion of the people who were interviewed. These were also the only items to show an increase in stigma over the study years.

There is little accessible evidence about the stigma of mental illnesses in other Asian countries, but it is probable that there are similarities between the cultural interpretation of mental illnesses found other Asian countries and those found in China. In Japan, for example, psychological distress is linked to personal weakness (such as a lack of willpower or self-control) and is, therefore, expressed in somatic terms. Beliefs about the hereditary and constitutional nature of mental illnesses lead to strong social stigmatization, including discrimination in marriage, business, and education, which may be experienced by both the patient and the family members. As family structures have become less extensive and more limited to the nuclear family, there has been an increasing reliance on mental hospitals so that the family may disassociate themselves from their ill relative. Once hospitalized, patients are discouraged from returning to their social

Table 3-1. PERCENT OF HONG KONG CHINESE IN AGREEMENT
(STRONGLY AGREE OR AGREE)

Questionnaire Item	1994 % of 2316	1996 % of 1273
Knowledge:		
Only a small portion of mental patients are violent or dangerous to others	74%	75%
Mental illness is not infectious or contagious	81%	86%
Most people would somehow experience mental health problems	65%	57%
Mental illness cannot be treated completely	17%	16%
Recovery Philosophy:		
Psychiatric rehabilitation facilities should be far from the community	44%	41%
Mental patients should best be kept in mental hospitals until they completely recover	55%	46%
Mental patients should not be kept in rehabilitation facilities other than mental hospitals	29%	27%
Social Distance:		
I do not want to live near any mental patients	44%	47%
I do not want to live near any psychiatric rehabilitation facilities	40%	43%

SOURCE: Kee Lee Chou, Ki-yan Mak. Attitudes to Mental Patients Among Hong Kong Chinese: A Trend Study Over Two Years. *Int J Soc Psychiatry* September 1998 44: 215–224. With permission from Sage.)

group. Similarly, in Southeast Asian cultures, mental illnesses are viewed as serious and untreatable. Having one's mental problems become known to others is a source of great shame and distress. Families will seek out indigenous healers and priests, rather than professional services. When one's illness is considered to be a result of bad behavior, social rejection is common. "Madness," which is considered untreatable, is highly stigmatized, though in some cultures, conditions that are acute and considered to be reversible—such as *Amok* in Malay culture (Arboleda-Flórez, 1979)—are viewed more tolerantly (Ng, 1997).

Griffiths and colleagues (2006) compared the nature and extent of stigma in Australia and Japan using a standardized household survey. Stigma was frequent in both countries, with item endorsements ranging from approximately 30% to 80%. Japanese respondents more frequently reported that a mentally ill person presented to them in a vignette could snap out of it if they wanted to, was suffering from a personal weakness, and did not have a medical illness. Japanese respondents were also less likely to report that they would hire such a person or vote for them in an election. Respondents in both countries expressed greater social distance for the vignette depicting someone with schizophrenia, compared to the vignette depicting someone with depression.

Furnham and Chan (2004) compared cultural differences between Hong Kong Chinese and British students with respect to lay theories of schizophrenia. British respondents were more apt to support a biological model of illness, whereas Chinese respondents supported a social-environmental (but not a superstitious) model. Chinese respondents held more negative attitudes toward people with schizophrenia, more often reporting that someone with schizophrenia was dangerous and uncontrollable. They believed that people with schizophrenia could lose control at any time and act outrageously in public places. They were more rejecting of the idea of building community-based treatment facilities near their homes and thought that people with schizophrenia should be kept segregated in distant mental hospitals.

Kurihara and colleagues (Kurihara, Kato, Sakamoto, Reverger, and Kitamura, 2000) noted some differences in the level of public stigma toward mental illnesses expressed between Balinese ($n = 77$) and Japanese samples ($n - 66$). They hypothesized that residents of Bali would be less prejudicial toward mental patients given that Bali was non-industrialized and had few psychiatric beds, suggesting a greater acceptance of people with a mental illness in the community. Using a measure designed to assess global levels of stigma in the community, the Balinese reported less stigma for persons with a history of psychiatric treatment. Levels of stigma varied in the two societies according to the type of mental illness, with Balinese participants expressing greater devaluation and discrimination towards persons with depressive and obsessive-compulsive disorders, and more positive attitudes towards people with schizophrenia. In Bali, disease is considered to be caused by an interaction known as *niskala* and *sekala*. The *sekala* component is the concrete aspect of the illness that can be removed by a physician. The *niskala* component is more abstract and considered to be better treated by a traditional healer. Most Balinese believe that psychotic disorders are caused by a *niskala* component, such as a supernatural phenomenon or black magic, so this may explain their less stigmatizing views of people with schizophrenia.

Indian Culture

Traditional Indian medical systems identify mental illnesses as distinct disorders. Treatments are provided by a range of practitioners, with no distinct setting or provider system predominating. Only with European colonization did separate mental health facilities emerge. As in most of Europe, "lunatic asylums" were segregated from population centers (Ganju, 2000).

There are at least three conceptually distinct medical traditions that are usually invoked to explain mental disorders: first, they are supposed to result from supernatural causes involving punishment by sorcery, gods, or spirits (traditional folk medicine); second, they arise from a disturbance of the normal healthy humoral balance (Ayurvedic medicine); and third, they stem from a dysfunction of the normal bio-psycho-social processes (modern medicine). These various interpretations of the etiology of mental illnesses give rise to a range of alternatives for treatment and management. Allopathic psychiatric services, Ayurvedic practitioners, homeopaths, folk healers, and healing temples are all recognized as options (Weiss, Sharma, Gaur, Sahrma, Desai, and Doongaji, 1986). In the rural areas of India, where over 80% of the population lives, modern psychiatry is absent. There, people rely on a variety of traditional healers, sometimes following the advice of more than one at a time. Where modern medicine is available, villagers consult both traditional healers and doctors, without this causing anxiety for the clients or the therapists (Kapur, 1979).

Serious mental illnesses are clearly distinguished from less serious forms. Chowdhury, Chakraborty, and Weiss (2001) studied local concepts of mental health in a rural area of West Bengal. Villagers considered madness (termed *Pagla* or *pagal*) to be characterized by talking nonsense and behaving in a hostile or aggressive manner. Assumed causes included diet, possession, traumatic shock, and smoking cannabis. In the early stages of the illness, the patient's family and friends would seek help from all available sources; however, if the disturbance did not improve quickly (traditional healers are often costly, so many families cannot afford treatment for a long time), families quickly lost hope and were known to abandon their ill relative. The term *pagal* is recognized throughout most of northern India, but the concept of *mental health* is not well understood.

A study of 101 consecutive patients with schizophrenia and family members who attended psychiatric clinic in Vellore, India, showed that the majority simultaneously held several and sometimes contradictory models of the illness and its treatment. Many of the patients had visited traditional healers, and three-quarters had used at least two systems of healing. Even though traditional models of illness are generally considered to be non-stigmatizing, those who endorsed models of illness that were based on karma and evil spirits reported higher stigma scores (Charles, Manoranjitham, and Jacob, 2007).

Despite the absence of a local term for *stigma* in many parts of India, stigma is a frequent experience among seriously ill patients. In a random sample of inpatients in Bangalore who had schizophrenia, most indicated they experienced shame and embarrassment (92%) and would keep others from knowing if possible (95%). Having schizophrenia would damage their prospects for marriage (98%) and would interfere with an existing marriage (95%). The majority also considered that others would think less of their family (70%); that they would refuse to visit the home (62%); and that it would cause problems for a relative to marry (87%). Family members were deeply ashamed of their relative's behavior and wished to keep them at home in an effort to conceal their illness and minimize negative implications for the other family members. Families felt blamed and were concerned their relatives who did not have schizophrenia would, nevertheless, pass it on to their children. Thus patients were kept at home, not only to conceal the condition, but to also conceal the perceived familial causes of the condition; which were a source of deep shame and embarrassment (Raguram, Raghu, Vounatsou, and Weiss, 2004). Similar findings have been reported in Chennai; with the addition that stigma was more often a concern when the patient was female, as difficulties with marriage prospects then loomed larger (Thara and Srinivasan, 2000).

As these various studies illustrate, the popular belief that traditional societies are more tolerant of people with mental illnesses because of religious and family ties is wrong. In addition, religious or magical views of mental illness may also carry significant connotations of moral or religious failure. Serious mental illnesses—those that are accompanied by disordered behavior—are considered particularly shameful and embarrassing. Confinement in hospitals away from the family would be the preferred solution so that the family could conceal the fact that they have a mentally relative in their midst. If hospitalization is not available, or families cannot afford treatments, people with a mental illness may find themselves ejected from their family life, turned into vagrants, and at high risk of death from starvation or violence.

4

Paradigm 3: Stigma Reduction Requires Well-Developed Plans

A CASE FOR ENLIGHTENED OPPORTUNISM

In this age of evidence-based policy and programming it may be anathema to suggest that long-term plans are not necessary for useful actions against stigma. However, traditional approaches to stigma reduction have been overly structured, top-down affairs. This makes it difficult to capitalize on local events as springboards to action, or involve local communities as active partners in anti-stigma activities. An alternate approach is to support individual and collective self-help and mutual aid efforts, thus creating a readiness to use opportunities, where they emerge, to effectively address problems related to stigma. From this perspective, the solution lies in building collaborative relationships among community stakeholders based on the shared value of creating local problem-solving capacities. The resulting community-based programs build on people's commitment to their own localities, provide opportunities for empowerment, and strengthen local relationships. Local stakeholders work together in ways that fit their own needs, and address local problems that they deem to be important. Even in the context of larger, national or international programs, local communities may still shape activities to fit their own needs and unique context (Florin and Wandersman, 1990).

In the old paradigm, programs typically directed generic messages about "mental illness" to the population at large using top-down educational and social-marketing approaches. Program messages and materials were developed to address perceived gaps in the public's knowledge; or to replace inaccurate and stereotypical portrayals with accurate information. Messages were typically developed by professional bodies to convey a scientific understanding of facts, such as the high prevalence of mental illnesses, that anyone can develop a mental illness, that those with a mental illness are not more dangerous than the rest of the population, or that mental illnesses are treatable. In some cases, mental health experts would provide lectures to target audiences, such as high school students or members of the general public, about the causes and consequences of mental illnesses. This traditional top-down approach addressed to the whole population assumes that development is a matter of catching up, transferring expert information, and creating technological fixes; but there is growing evidence that it does not work. Despite some improvements in public knowledge and attitudes over time, there remains clear evidence of the public's desire to keep people with a mental illness at bay by excluding them from social relationships (Angermeyer and Dietrich, 2006), and education about the causes of mental disorders may increase this social distance (Sartorius, 2010).

In 1996, when international experts were convened to help plan the World Psychiatric Association's *Open the Doors* anti-stigma initiative, much consideration went into developing a set of specific plans that were to be applied in all participating countries and offered to national action groups to help them outline the activities they should undertake and estimate the timelines associated with these. However, consultations with national action groups quickly showed that a different strategy was needed—one that was tailored to fit their local circumstances and allowed members to take advantage of important local opportunities as they arose. While the new strategy seemed, at first, to be dangerously similar to a plan for wholesale confusion, it quickly became the hallmark of the program and one of its most important features. Rather than planning from the top down, a bottom-up approach was used; one that relied heavily on the experiences of those who were most closely associated with the consequences of stigma, as well as those who were most strategically positioned to provide community-level support for anti-stigma activities (Sartorius and Schulze, 2005).

The recognition of local contexts stands out as one of the key tasks of programs that aim to bring about community change. Development initiatives that build on local issues and galvanize local interest and experience are more likely to be effective. Also, by participating and consolidating community action, people who are marginalized can reclaim their position in their social group, reaffirm their identities and social worth, and become active participants in community-level interventions (Campbell and Jovchelovitch, 2000). Florin and Wandersman (1990) have noted that isolating social problems and assigning them to a large or bureaucratic institution to "fix" increasingly results in frustration. However, individual and collective mutual aid efforts that are coordinated and supported by a formal system have shown much greater results. These typically form around organizations that are locally situated, volunteer-driven, with broad participation from people who share a mutual interest in solving a problem. While some support is required to maintain functions, typically funding is on a much smaller scale, and in some cases nonexistent.

Top-down approaches are cumbersome and inefficient because they often fail to recognize and harness local resources. They do not pay attention to local realities and they do not integrate local systems of knowledge and action. Consequently, they are perceived by those most directly concerned—people with a mental illness and their families—as being "foreign" and imposed, and so tend to be ineffective. In recent years, health-promotion efforts focusing on health inequalities have shifted emphasis from top-down interventions (which often only give lip service to participation) to a community-development perspective. This perspective is based on the idea that health programs are likely to have an impact only if they are built to satisfy the local needs, follow the local situation, and involve members of the communities in their planning and implementation. People are far more likely to change their behaviors when local leaders and trusted peers are involved in the design and implementation of local programs directed to problems that people with a mental illness and their family members see as important. Thus, health promoters are increasingly involved in community-strengthening programs that try to create enabling communities characterized by trust, mutual support, and high levels of involvement. Approaches that build on local contexts and representations are likely to be seen as more relevant and therefore more sustainable (Campbell and Jovchelovitch, 2000).

We use the term *enlightened opportunism* to reflect the readiness of grassroots groups to use windows of opportunity as springboards for targeted local action. We contrast enlightened opportunism with the conventional program-planning paradigm that would require a clear, *a priori* path to be charted between specific program activities, in a specific order, and with long-term (distal) outcomes. Anti-stigma programs that use enlightened opportunism are fluid and flexible. Their activities use windows of opportunities and are embedded in, and responsive to local communities.

To consider that the stigma attached to mental illnesses can best be reduced through well-structured, long-term programs portrays anti-stigma programming as a highly structured, technical activity that must be reserved for people with expert skills, and overlooks the impact that all individuals may make through smaller, focused actions that may be taken during the course of their day-to-day lives. A key strength of the model of enlightened opportunism is that anyone and everyone can take advantage of opportunities to improve social inclusion for people with a mental illness—either through direct personal action or by supporting others. Also, in most locations, outside of large, nationally funded programs, the bulk of resources for anti-stigma activities are volunteered. Voluntary organizations, particularly if they involve a widely spread membership, are vulnerable, and some studies report that half fail in the first year (Florin and Wandersman, 1990). Grassroots initiatives have a better

chance of surviving, because they meet the common interests of the participants and do not depend on a single key individual who may burn out over
time. Programs are also virtually guaranteed to fail if their goals appear to be
too futuristic or unachievable. Anti-stigma programs must last a long time if
they are to be successful. A major obstacle to their long duration is that those
who lead them tire and burn out. Measurable "quick wins" are an important
antidote this development because they renew enthusiasm and maintain the
momentum of the work (Sartorius, 2006).

NETWORKS OF PRACTICE

In the last ten years, the business and managerial literature has shown a growing interest in the idea of developing and sharing knowledge through networks
of practice. The emergence of network societies focusing on complex development goals—such as eliminating stigma attributed to mental illnesses—represents a new paradigm in development thinking (Murdoch, 2000). *Networks* are
self-managing systems whose members have common values and who share
trust, knowledge, and working practices. They are highly fluid and depend on
the ongoing social relationships that have been established between members
to promote collective action (Baker, Kan, and Teo, 2011)

Practice networks have been described as the core of socially situated learning.
In a socially situated view of learning, individuals continuously combine and
modify context-specific knowledge to create collective expertise (Tagliaventi
and Mattarelli, 2006). When networks focus on development goals, they have
the opportunity to straddle spaces, to draw on outside expertise, and to solve
more complex problems. The *Open the Doors* program used "Local Action
Groups" to form the core of community-based anti-stigma work and then net-
worked these globally, using a range of activities including face-to-face social
activities, meetings at scientific conferences, a web page, and an electronic chat
space (Sartorius and Schulze, 2005).

Unlike large bureaucratic organizations, networks of practice are borderless
and flexible, making them particularly well suited to anti-stigma work that
uses a model of enlightened opportunism to guide program activities. They
can change quickly and invent new structures and activities that are responsive to members' interests as well as to local circumstances and opportunities.
New members may be quickly enlisted when required to address emerging
opportunities, which fosters sustainability. Networks also provide an important training ground. They build collaboration, consensus, and continuous
learning. Collaborative relationships build trust, which is essential for the
development of new ideas and approaches. Successful networks are flexible,

responsive to their members, and continually learning and reinventing themselves. Networks lend themselves to diversity of partners and multi-agency involvement. Also, enabling members to create and sustain network partnerships and to participate in advancing the goals of the network is empowering (Liberman, 2000).

Many positive outcomes stem from the sense of community that is generated by a practice network, strong feelings of commitment to shared goals, availability of support, cooperation among members, satisfaction with group activities, and improved flow of information among network members. Networks also promote collaborative group learning, which occurs through interaction, evaluation, and cooperation. Network members learn through critical reflection about the problems they have faced, the roadblocks that may have slowed their activities, and from interventions that have had unexpected effects. Sharing experiences and solutions creates a sense of joint enterprise. Members can draw on each other's knowledge and experiences and become more effective at solving problems. Exposure to alternate points of view can challenge and motivate. Tools and solutions developed in one part of the network can be quickly disseminated among all of the partners, thus eliminating the need to continually start from scratch (Benbunan-Fich and Hiltz, 1999). Activities of specific members may ebb and flow, but the network will maintain a sense of momentum (Sartorius and Schulze, 2005). A key factor that supports the sustainability of network activities is that the network remains open to newcomers and allows them to move from peripheral status, in their role as newcomer, to more central roles, including leadership roles. The network must be able to draw in new participants on an ongoing basis without disrupting activities where longer-standing members can mentor newer members (Wegerif, 1998). Our experience has shown that teaching by persons who have conducted successful programs is more credible, is better remembered, and can more easily lead to action.

NETWORK GOVERNANCE AND LEADERSHIP

Baker et al. (2011) described three types of governance structures that have been identified in the network literature: shared governance; lead organization governance; and administrative governance (when one organization has been specifically designated to oversee the network, and all activities and decisions are coordinated through it). Networks that are formally constructed are more likely to fail.

Networks that are informally constructed emerge out of prior relationships. Their successful evolution is often dependent on individual players. A strong, visionary leader may unite network partners under a unified vision, empower them, and provide a participatory environment in which to address network objectives. The most effective leaders are those who focus on people-oriented behaviors, in addition to the tasks at hand; foster communication between network partners; and nurture a unifying vision. Maintaining a unifying vision is particularly important when network partners represent autonomous organizations.

Goodman and colleagues (1998) have identified ten dimensions of leadership that they consider important for community development work:

- Inclusion of formal and informal leaders;
- Providing direction and structure for participants;
- Encouraging participation from a diverse network of community participants;
- Implementing procedures to insure participation from all during group meetings and events;
- Facilitating the sharing of information and resources;
- Shaping and cultivating new leaders;
- A responsive and accessible style;
- The ability to focus on both task and process details;
- Receptivity to prudent innovation and risk taking; and
- Connectedness to other leaders.

When considering who will lead, it is important to distinguish between *positional* leaders (those who occupy leadership positions by appointment or election) and *reputational* leaders (those who have served the community in informal leadership capacities, such as activists or other opinion leaders who serve as norm-setters). In Chapter 6, we will argue that mental health professionals should not assume that they will be the *de facto* leaders of anti-stigma efforts by virtue of their position or their agency. Anti-stigma activities can best be served by grassroots leaders who are respected in the local community for their contributions to mental health advocacy and who are capable of providing a democratic style of leadership that empowers network partners. Otherwise, program activities may become a process of social and political control.

Hailey and James (2004) describe "development leaders" who have a clear vision, a firm set of values, and a strong sense of commitment to helping marginalized groups. They are described as pragmatic; willing to apply new technologies and draw on science or other sources of applied professional knowledge, and they have an ability to analyze the external environment for emerging trends and opportunities. They can adapt to different roles and needs, and have the capacity to combine ideals and values with analysis, technical expertise, and professionalism. They balance diverse demands and personal commitments with the needs of local communities, vested interests of local pressure groups, and the demands of funders.

GENERAL PRINCIPLES, RATHER THAN SPECIFIC PLANS, GUIDE ANTI-STIGMA ACTIVITIES

Detailed, *a priori*, long-term specific plans are not necessary to guide anti-stigma activities. However, in order to make maximum use of enlightened opportunism and foster strong networks of practice, it is important to have a shared vision. As well as helping to create a sense of community within network partners, having general principles to guide activities aids in deciding which emergent opportunities are appropriate to pursue and which should be bypassed. We have found the following six principles to be a useful starting point for anti-stigma activities:

1. **Put people first:** People who have a mental illness, and their family members, must be central in the process of stigma reduction. They must be the ones to set the targets for change, and they must be involved as equal partners in every level of planning, programming, and evaluation. Not only will this provide the program with targets that are meaningful, it will offer opportunities for social interaction, empowerment, and local change. While the process of stigmatization plays out in similar ways, the specific issues that may impede or bother people will be locally driven. In order to aim for real change in the lives of people who experience stigma, it is important to understand the local context by asking those who are most directly affected. In most parts of the world, there is no research that documents the personal impact of stigma, either in terms of the frequency of occurrence or of the impact of stigmatizing experiences. Without this information, anti-stigma programs run the risk of developing goals and objectives that are misaligned to the real problems. Anti-stigma programs that are grounded in the day-to-day experiences of people who have a mental illness and their family members stand the best chance of success.

2. **Plan for sustainability:** The social processes that produce stigma related to mental illnesses are complex, pervasive, and mutually reinforcing— all characteristics that are resistant to change. This means that programs against stigma must take the long view and plan for sustainability from the outset. Program developers must resist the temptation to frame their

activities in terms of campaigns, which typically involve short bursts of activity that do not create sustained change. To be successful, anti-stigma programs must last. Often, anti-stigma programs are poorly funded, so rely on volunteer resources coupled with an occasional infusion of funds. This means that anti-stigma programs must retain the loyalty of supporters and consider ways in which new generations of workers will be recruited, trained, and moved into leadership positions. Having tools and toolkits will help newcomers to the program continue along a planned course of action.

3. **Focus on activities that change behaviors:** In Chapters 7 and 8, we will argue that there is no clear relationship between knowledge, attitudes, and behavioral change, particularly when dealing with deep-seated preju-dices. Therefore, considering improvements in knowledge or attitudes as of evidence of future behavior-change is problematic. In order to bring about meaningful improvement for people who experience stigma, sig-nificant behavioral change must occur. This should include changes at the individual level in carefully targeted groups, combined with changes in the way organizations behave. Multipronged programs that approach a targeted behavioral change from different levels—individual, group, and organizational—have a better chance of bringing about meaningful change. Indicators of success of anti-stigma programs must also be directly related to behavioral change, such as the enactment of anti-discrimination legislation, higher re-employment rates, fewer difficulties in finding safe and affordable housing, or reduced bullying in the schools.

4. **Target activities to well-defined groups:** A corollary of the third prin-ciple that focuses on behavioral change is that anti-stigma activities tar-geting specific behaviors or a special subgroup of the population (such as judges, teachers, or health staff) have a better chance of changing behavior and are more likely to be successful.

5. **Think big, but start small:** The long-term goal of every anti-stigma program must be to eliminate discrimination experienced by people with a mental illness in order to promote their full and effective participation in valued social roles and relationships. Toward these ends, small successes go a long way, both in terms of reaffirming that stigma can be beaten, and in terms of maintaining the enthusiasm of all participants—those from relevant service agencies, people with a mental illness, their family mem-bers, and other volunteers. This means that programs must seize impor-tant opportunities for success whenever they present themselves. The

accumulation and celebration of "quick wins" will create and maintain program momentum and avoid burnout. It is also important to communicate successes to local funders, program planners, local media, and other constituents, as these will provide an important source of positive news and may help generate much-needed funding. On a larger scale, this principle also holds for the development of comprehensive national programs: they must be the final outcome of numerous local programs that are directed to local problems and are successful in overcoming them.

6. **Build Better Practices:** Building better practices is all about learning from mistakes, which every program will make. Critical reflection, systematic evaluation, and a spirit of inquiry will help in this regard. It is also important to build on the work of others—to understand the active ingredients and to have a clear idea which components of programs require modification to make them appropriate for local conditions. Documentation of these is also essential. Because the best practices that catch the eye of funders and policy makers are those culled from the scientific literature, it is important to insure that experience is translated into systematic evaluations whose results find their way to decision-makers, to the lay public, and into peer-reviewed publications. This means that anti-stigma programs will want to partner with local evaluators and researchers to ensure that they have sound evaluation methods and the expertise to make sure that results are published and widely disseminated.

Community-based programs hold considerable promise for the reduction or eradication of stigma. The process of gaining control through participating with others to change social and political realities is an important empowerment strategy for people who have a mental illness and their family members. This is one of the reasons why they must be central to any anti-stigma effort; another being that it is only through their continuous collaboration that the program can remain focused on problems that are the most disturbing for people who have a mental illness and for their family members. To be successful, anti-stigma programs must practice enlightened opportunism, as this will allow them to capitalize on important local initiatives and accrue successes. Programs must remain flexible and nimble, or they will be unable to take advantage of opportunities as they present themselves. Because the eradication of stigma is a long-term goal, programs must also consider their own sustainability. Developing networks of practice among a variety of local stakeholders and programs is a useful strategy for meeting all of these goals.

5

Paradigm 4: Science Is the Best Guide

for Programmes

EVIDENCE-BASED ADVOCACY

A key assumption of the current paradigm governing anti-stigma work is that scientifically collected data, rather than subjective beliefs or personal wants, will be the yardstick against which funding priorities will be measured and program effectiveness will be judged. The important premise is that evidence-based policy and practice will eliminate potentially discriminatory variations in practice, remove political influence as a determinant of program worth, and ultimately lead to greater fairness and equity in service delivery. It is also predicted that evidence demonstrating the effectiveness of stigma-reduction programs will boost confidence among funders that such programs are worthy of their financial attention and make it increasingly difficult for policy makers to defend policies that disadvantage people with a mental illness (Stuart, 2009).

Unfortunately, program targets chosen on the basis of scientific evidence often have no resonance among people who have a mental illness, their family members, or local constituencies. As the effects of stigma may be experienced in many ways, local conditions and priorities will be the most useful guides in defining which consequences of stigma are the most burdensome and might, therefore, deserve priority in an action program. Even when research in an area has identified a serious problem, local anti-stigma action groups may not wish to focus on that problem, given local circumstances. It may be too politically intractable and divert energies away from areas where early successes seem more probable. Therefore, scientific knowledge, where it exists, can be only one of the factors that should be taken into account in deciding on program goals and methods of work.

A second problem with evidence-based advocacy is that it postulates that targets should be chosen on the basis of evidence that an effective intervention exists. From this perspective, needs are defined on the basis of an ability to effectively intervene. Unfortunately, the growing interest in stigma, and a resulting cottage industry in stigma-reduction programs, has not been paralleled by a similar interest in program evaluation. Few anti-stigma programs have been rigorously evaluated. The scientific evidence, though growing, remains meager and is insufficient to authoritatively establish "best practices" in the field of stigma reduction. A number of promising practices have been identified, but few have been implemented widely enough to understand their broad public health benefits, sustainability, or costs. Therefore, there is too little evidence about the effectiveness of anti-stigma interventions to guide program selection, particularly where large population groups are concerned.

Finally, a related problem is that the preferred methods for generating scientific evidence are poorly suited to this field, as they favor interventions that can be studied using conventional experiments (such as randomized controlled trials) or syntheses of studies using experimental approaches. Because anti-stigma interventions are oriented toward bringing about community-level or organizational change, they are often not amenable to validation using experimental approaches. Thus, for example, anti-stigma interventions aimed at changing social and organizational structures in workplaces are more amenable to case studies, organizational ethnographies, or other qualitative approaches. Some anti-stigma programs target entire nations and populations, making them more suited to quasi-experimental and observational designs—evidence that is usually considered by scientists to be of lower quality and so excluded from systematic reviews (Stuart, 2008).

EVIDENCE IS IN THE EYE OF THE BEHOLDER

Like beauty or art, "evidence" is in the eye of the beholder. Particularly in an applied field, the nature and quality of the "evidence" that is used by program developers to make program decisions can vary widely. Thus, one challenge in bringing researchers and community partners together to develop and implement anti-stigma programs is bridging the different knowledge cultures. Community agencies rarely have opportunities for in-depth monitoring, reflection, and learning. They cannot afford to invest in formal research, either as consumers or as producers, but instead need knowledge that is contextualized, easily accessible, decision-oriented, and pragmatic. Thus, they accept a much broader range of evidence and share it much more informally. Academics, on the other hand, pursue formal, objective knowledge that has been de-contextualized and carefully cross-examined following a lengthy peer-review process

(Ferguson, 2005). In addition, different cultures, and groups within cultures, view knowledge and evidence quite differently.

The question of how much each side should compromise its view of "evidence" for purposes of policy and program development is a thorny one—one that may not be so easily solved in the mental health field, with its longstanding disciplinary and ideological divisions. Evidence-informed decision making entails finding a way to synthesize the formal scientific evidence of research with the colloquial wisdom and knowledge of practice. Lomas (2006) argues that the compromise as to what counts as "evidence" cannot fall to one side or the other. Rather, the way forward is to give up our historical drive to fit science into decision-making, and find new ways of incorporating pragmatic, colloquial knowledge into science.

In the pursuit of anti-stigma programming, another community of knowledge—the lived experiences of people who are stigmatized—must be heavily represented. This includes people who have a mental illness, as well as their family members and care providers. Personal stories, testimonials, and qualitative reports must all be factored into the evidence equation. To date, the bulk of stigma theory and research has failed to be informed by the lived experiences of those who are stigmatized (Link and Phelan, 2001).

To avoid the false assumptions that may result from failing to incorporate experiential evidence, it is important for local anti-stigma teams to base program development and the selection of program targets on knowledge of the day-to-day experiences of those who are stigmatized (Sartorius, 2004). The German *Open the Doors* team (Schulze and Angermeyer, 2003) conducted a focus-group study of patients with schizophrenia, their relatives, and mental health professionals. This study found that stigma experiences went far beyond direct personal contact with others—the focus of much of the current research. In particular, stigma was experienced through structural imbalances built into legal regulations, health insurance statutes, and political decisions, as well as through the largely negative media portrayals of mental illness. A second important finding was that patients, family members, and mental health providers, while in agreement with the broad dimensions of stigma, attached different priorities to each of these areas. These differences underscore the importance of including patient and family experiences when setting anti-stigma targets.

TO BE SUCCESSFUL, PROGRAMS MUST TARGET LOCAL NEEDS

Although the stigma attached to mental illnesses is universal, it plays out in locally specific ways. The experience of someone with schizophrenia in Egypt is not that of someone in the United States. It seems fundamental, therefore, that anti-stigma programs should be designed to meet the local needs of people who experience stigma and discrimination. Our experience has been that scientific knowledge, which by definition is designed to be generalizable, is rarely helpful in determining these designs.

Even though science may not be helpful in defining local targets, scientific methods are. Anti-stigma groups must approach the task of assessing needs in a systematic manner, using a combination of qualitative and quantitative methods to explore the personal experiences and priorities of people who have a mental illness, and those of their family members. In this respect, a *situational analysis* is a helpful tool. A situational analysis is a systematic investigation of a complex problem that impacts people and systems. It offers a method for selecting program targets that is rigorous and evidence-informed. It is well suited to anti-stigma activities because it is consultative and collaborative, and it recognizes and values multiple stakeholder views. It encourages engagement from people who have local knowledge, and it results in a clear sense of direction and practice. Most important, it allows for the integration of collective knowledge of participants into the strategic decision making process. The resulting contextualized knowledge provides an enriched perspective on whatever scientific evidence exists and should be seen as complementary (Ammam, 2005).

Following a situational analysis, the local action team will have a long list of issues and potential interventions. The list can then be categorized into issues that pertain to stigma and those that pertain to other factors. Program members can then sift through the list of stigma-related issues to identify which ones will be the targets for the anti-stigma program. Anti-stigma groups should pick issues assiduously, based on the probability that they can be addressed using the combined expertise of the network partners that have been recruited; that there are sufficient resources (including political influence) to address the problem; and perhaps most important, that there are sufficient opportunities for early successes. Once targets are known, reference to the scientific literature and experience from other anti-stigma programs may inform intervention approaches.

TO BE SUCCESSFUL, PROGRAMS MUST BUILD BETTER PRACTICES

Though scholarly interest in anti-stigma programming and evaluation is increasing, the evidence base supporting best practices in the field remains underdeveloped and insufficient to support the growing interest in stigma reduction. A review of applied-health literature using databases such as OVID,

Medline, and PsychInfo shows little applied interest in stigma attached to mental illnesses until the middle of the 1990s. Since that time, the number of articles pertaining to mental health and mental illnesses with the key terms *stigma* or *discrimination* in the title or abstract has grown, but still remains less than 2% of all publications (Stuart, 2008). It also should be noted that the bulk of the publications are from industrialized countries. Figure 5.1 shows the number of articles published in peer-reviewed journals in the PsychInfo database between 2000 and November 2011 with the word *stigma* in the title.

One impetus for building better practices for anti-stigma programs comes from the rise of evidence-based practice in general, whose goal is to reduce unjustified variations in outcomes, promote safe and efficacious interventions, and reduce the time needed to incorporate scientifically sound results into best-practice standards of care (Haynes, 2002). Evidence about the time that it takes to achieve goals is important because early successes are needed for anti-stigma programs to maintain momentum and convince community stakeholders that stigma can be beaten. To be incorporated into best-practice approaches, program successes must be systematically documented as part of ongoing system-monitoring and evaluation. Thus, the impetus for ongoing evaluation draws momentum from a desire to critically assess processes and outcomes, to learn from mistakes, and to assure one another that the burden of suffering has been diminished and not inadvertently magnified. It is something that we undertake for ourselves—based on our desire to learn and to be accountable to network partners and funders—rather than something that is imposed from without (Scriven, 1991).

Policy makers and funders in many countries face unprecedented pressure to support their decisions with scientific evidence of program effectiveness (Black, 2001). Because the evidence base supporting anti-stigma programming is still in its infancy, careful ongoing evaluation of anti-stigma initiatives is necessary to contribute new understanding about the causal mechanisms underlying successful planning and to ensure that successful programs are reproducible. A

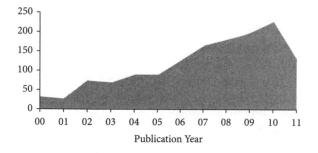

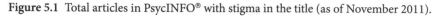

Figure 5.1 Total articles in PsycINFO® with stigma in the title (as of November 2011).

clear demonstration that anti-stigma interventions are having the desired effect will build momentum for local activities, create confidence in program partners, and help convince local funders that stigma can be beaten and that anti-stigma activities deserve to be funded. Evidence-hungry policy makers and funders will use the *lack* of evidence to restrict funding opportunities for anti-stigma programs. In this climate, unambiguous findings supporting better practices that have been produced by rigorous evaluations will be an important advocacy tool. Not only will evidence supporting effectiveness be instrumental in diverting funding and resources to anti-stigma programs, it will make it increasingly difficult for future decision-makers to defend policies and practices that systematically disadvantage people with a mental illness (Stuart, 2008).

Building better- and best-practices in anti-stigma programming will require program networks to clearly understand and articulate the principles and procedures underlying their program activities in ways that will allow them to be meaningfully tested using a variety of research methods and techniques. Understanding why a programs works, or does not work, will be as important as demonstrating that it produces the right kind of change. Only by understanding why an intervention is likely to work and by articulating and testing its various assumptions will it be possible to build generalizable theories of change. In addition to achieving good results locally, it will be critical to be able to clearly specify the "active ingredients" so that they can be replicated in other locations. Theory-based evaluation challenges program providers to make their program assumptions explicit; to link these to available scientific knowledge (if it exists); and then to assess which of these hold, which break down, and why. Once this is known, activities and resources can be concentrated on the activities that are most powerful in reducing the stigma attached to mental illnesses. Programs that adopt this approach will be more policy-relevant because they will contribute new knowledge that is generalizable (Weiss, 1995).

Anti-stigma programmers may confront difficult issues when creating better practices, such as the unbridled enthusiasm of volunteers and advocates, and the difficulties that sometimes occur when trying to curb the desire to act, rather than reflect. Having a clearly developed planning process that includes an *a priori* evaluation strategy, such as the one articulated by the *Open the Doors* anti-stigma program, can help channel energies and initial enthusiasms into these important activities. Ultimately, building better practices in anti-stigma programming will depend on building bridges between scientific and practitioner communities and worldviews.

In conclusion, scientific evidence may not help anti-stigma groups choose important targets, because these must be locally relevant and achievable—something that scientific evidence cannot address. Second, there is the presupposition that interventions must be based on best practices, as represented in the scientific literature. This may not be possible, because the literature dealing with best practices in anti-stigma programming is meager and may not be helpful to programs that are developing novel approaches, or those that want to use the experiences of other existing programs. When scientific evidence exists, it can be used to inform delivery options. More often however, programs will need to implement their own evaluative processes to systematically collect and interpret outcome data in order to build an evidence base for anti-stigma activities.

6

Paradigm 5: Psychiatrists Should Lead Antistigma Programmes

MENTAL HEALTH PROFESSIONALS ARE WORTHY TARGETS OF ANTI-STIGMA PROGRAMS

Psychiatrists and other health and social service professions often expect to lead community based anti-stigma programs because they consider that their advanced education in psychiatry and related disciplines will have equipped them with the requisite knowledge and skills. They may doubt the competency of lay people, or people who have experienced a mental illness, to conduct such programs. Their working assumption often is that they exercise power on behalf of their client communities and learn about client needs through surveys and other community assessment techniques that are designed to rise above the clamor of vested interests. Against this backdrop, advocacy groups are often viewed as a problem, rather than a resource—asking for things that the professionals may consider unrealistic. On the other hand, ongoing service inadequacies, periodic funding cuts, and more general social inequities may give service-users little confidence that their opinions will be heard or that their concerns will carry weight. People in marginalized groups must expend a considerable amount of effort to find ways of collaborating with professionals (O'Keefe and Hogg, 1999).

A second problem is that many mental health professionals and mental health service systems have perpetuated stigma and fostered social exclusion. This makes them part of the problem and undermines their ability to generate trust. Many people who have received mental health services do not speak highly of the mental health professionals, who are often rated, ironically, as being among the most stigmatizing of all groups (Thornicroft, Rose, and Mehta, 2010). Recurrent themes include feeling punished, patronized, humiliated, spoken to as if they were children, being excluded from decisions, and being assumed to lack the capacity to be responsible for their own lives. Other problems include not being given sufficient information about their condition and treatment options, and feeling an unspoken threat of coercive treatment: which may be overt in instances of mandated care (in forensic psychiatry or civil-commitment proceedings). Mental health professionals are often unaware of the various facets of their own behaviors that add to the stigmatization process. In working with different mental health–related professional groups, we have often been told that stigma is an important issue, but also that "WE don't stigmatize our clients." Mental health professionals often feel entirely blameless. Stigma is something that "other people" do. Rather than being leaders of anti-stigma interventions, then, they are worthy targets of such programs.

The discriminatory and stigmatizing views held by health and mental health professionals have been largely ignored in attitude research. In qualitative studies, people with mental illnesses report considerable stigmatization from their mental health providers. They also deem the poor quality of mental health services to be discriminatory. The situation is even worse in developing countries where mental health services are underdeveloped, largely institutionally based, and lacking even elementary community supports. As well as being an antitherapeutic and highly negative experience, having an admission into such an institution will mark a patient and the family for life.

In their focus-group study in Germany, Schulze and Angermeyer (2003) found that stigma associated with mental health care accounted for one-quarter of all stigmatizing experiences reported by people with schizophrenia and their family members. People also felt discriminated against by mental health providers' lack of interest in them as a person, and the prognostic negativity with which their psychiatric diagnoses were given. Cavalier use of medications with socially important side-effects, such as weight gain and extrapyramidal symptoms, complicated their social interactions and reduced their self-esteem. They expressed the feeling that they were reduced to their illness-related deficits and were disheartened by the messages that they would be ill for the rest of their lives or were likely to commit suicide.

In a qualitative study focusing on 15 leaders of peer-support mental health programs (those provided by people who have themselves experienced a mental illness), "paternalism" was identified as a key barrier to recovery because it limited their ability to develop identities outside of their diagnostic label. Many participants reported that their mental health professional had told them that they would never recover; would never be able to work; would never go to school; would never be able to engage in challenging activities; and would never be a parent. In one extreme example, a nurse forced a patient, who was making notes about the subculture of the ward for a school project, to relinquish her student identity by publicly stating to the ward: *I am a mental patient. I am not a student* (Mancini, Hardiman, and Lawson, 2005, p. 51).

In Australia, Caldwell and Jorm (2001) examined beliefs about the prognosis and long-term outcomes of depression or schizophrenia. Only 2% of psychiatrists thought that, with professional help, someone with schizophrenia would make a full recovery, compared to 9% of mental health nurses, 3% of clinical psychologists, 3% of general practitioners—and 30% of the general public. With respect to depression, 37% of psychiatrists thought that someone with depression would make a full recovery with no further problems, compared to 42% mental health nurses, 45% of clinical psychologists, 24% of general practitioners, and 47% of the general public. Psychiatrists were the least optimistic of any group. Allied mental health professionals and general practitioners were considerably more pessimistic in their prognosis than were members of the general public. Having predetermined negative prognostic beliefs undermines recovery, encourages patients to adopt negative views, and lowers expectations—a pessimism that may grow with age and experience. Similar results have been reported elsewhere (Hugo, 2001), suggesting that mental health providers need to be more aware of their attitudes and careful about the expectations for recovery that they convey to their patients and family caregivers. Similarly, in Switzerland, Lauber and colleagues (2006) compared the stereotypes held by psychiatrists to those of other mental health professionals and the general population. Compared to other professional groups (psychologists, nurses, and other therapists), psychiatrists held more stigmatizing views. They considered people with a mental illness as more dangerous, less skilled, and more socially disturbing. Despite their greater clinical knowledge, mental health professionals held attitudes similar to the general population's with respect to key stereotypes, such as dangerousness and unpredictability.

Mental health professionals tend to base their views on their personal experiences working with people who have mental illnesses, with the majority of these experiences reflecting times when people are unwell, giving them a biased view of mental illnesses and the possibility of recovery. It is important to remember that people who recover from their mental illness do not maintain ties with the service system, and in order to avoid stigma, they may not speak about their illness or its successful treatment. As a result, many mental health practitioners will have a biased view of the true success of their interventions, the course and prognoses of many mental illnesses, and of the recovery process itself, because they only see patients who do not recover or who have relapsed, and seldom see those who are successfully managing their illness (Thornicroft, 2006). This situation challenges the strategy of using psychiatrists, or any mental health professional, as opinion leaders or as role models in anti-stigma interventions. They also indicate that mental health professionals must gain greater awareness of their own stereotypical views and how these may influence therapeutic goals.

STIGMA IN GENERAL HEALTH-CARE SETTINGS

An estimated three-quarters of those with a psychiatric diagnosis will receive care in general-practice settings. The prevalence of mental illness among patients attending general-practice settings has been estimated to be 25% to 30%, though half of these individuals will go undetected (Carr, Lewin, Walton, Faehrmann, and Reid, 1997; Ustun and Sartorius, 1995). In addition to people who contact health-service providers because of symptoms of their mental illness, a physician or nurse will regularly come into contact with patients who have a mental disorder comorbid to a physical illness. Among medical inpatients, for example, the prevalence of mental illnesses ranges between 30% and 40%, though medical nurses and doctors detect only about half of these (Hansen, Fink, Frydenberg, Oxhoj, Sondergaard, and Munk-Jorgensen, 2001).

People with a mental illness and their families report experiencing stigma in general medical settings where they have been treated with a lack of dignity, and sometimes with outright contempt. In a series of focus groups conducted in the United Kingdom, service users most often mentioned family doctors as a group that should be targeted for anti-stigma interventions (Thornicroft, Rose, and Mehta, 2010). In these settings, *diagnostic overshadowing* (the process by which physical symptoms are misattributed to a mental illness) was a barrier to receiving appropriate medical care. *Treatment overshadowing* describes a more generic bias that may influence treatment decisions. Diagnostic and treatment overshadowing may result from a host of factors, including clinicians' lack of knowledge about mental illnesses, their discomfort in dealing with people who have a mental illness, and their stigmatizing attitudes (Jones, Howard, and Thornicroft, 2008). In addition, they may misattribute the risk associated with certain medical procedures when applied to people who have a mental illness, so fail to offer these as possible treatment options.

Studies have shown that medical training may do little to improve students' negative attitudes toward people with a mental illness. In a study conducted in Turkey, students in their final year of medical education expressed a level of social distance toward someone described in a depression vignette that was comparable to that of students in their first year. Half the medical students expressed concern about having contact with the person described in the vignette—significantly more than comparison subjects who attended engineering school, or members of a public education center. Final-year medical students were less optimistic about the possibility of recovery and were more likely to indicate that hospitalization was required (Inandi, Aydin, Turhan, and Gultekin, 2008).

Nurses have also been identified as holding negative and pejorative beliefs. In a recent review of the nursing literature, Ross and Goldner (2009) found that nurses held many of the same stereotypical beliefs as the general public, particularly around attributions of dangerousness and unpredictability. In many of the studies reviewed, nurses disclosed that they lacked the skills to confidently and competently manage behavioral symptoms. Nurses' attitudes were particularly hostile toward people who required treatment for self-harm, and these individuals were perceived as squandering precious health-care resources intended to preserve life. Emergency room nurses and those in intensive care units were among the most hostile toward patients who had self-harmed and were often reported to be disrespectful and demeaning. Lack of clinical knowledge about the causes of suicide was widespread, and there was a belief that dealing with the mental-health components of care was "not their job"; that they had better and more constructive things to do. These attitudes were found despite professional rhetoric championing caring values, holistic care, health promotion, and advocacy. Mental health nurses, though often reported to be more accepting and less hostile than general medical nurses, also demonstrated negative attitudes and discriminatory treatment, particularly toward patients with a borderline personality disorder. These clients were viewed as difficult, annoying, manipulative, and attention-seeking, and were labeled with offensive terms such as *time-wasters* or *frequent flyers*. Rather than being perceived as *ill*, they were perceived as *bad*, with the result that nurses' communications with them were disparaging and unempathetic. Mental health nurses also held more pessimistic views about prognosis than the general public, leading them to give discouraging information and convey a sense of hopelessness to clients and families.

MENTAL HEALTH SYSTEMS AS AGENTS OF SOCIAL CONTROL

Asylums were originally built to protect people with a mental illness from the members of their communities (hence the term *asylum*). In time, they replaced jails and poorhouses as mechanisms of social control for members of society who were deemed to be too disruptive or inconvenient to have living in the community. In those early days, mental health systems, particularly psychiatrists, occupied a dual role—on one hand providing restorative interventions, and on the other, institutionalizing those who were deemed to be dangerous or disruptive to society, and exercising this power through civil-commitment and criminal proceedings with few due-process safeguards.

Social changes in the practice of psychiatry resulting from changes to civil-commitment legislation and the reduction in the number of psychiatric beds have meant that only those with the highest risk of violence against themselves or others receive treatment in inpatient settings. From early declarations disavowing the competence of mental health professionals to predict violence (Steadman, 1972), mental health professionals and systems have become increasingly geared toward the identification and management of dangerousness. Risk-management tools have emerged, and the prediction of violence is increasingly promoted as a core mental health skill—something that is expected of mental health providers and prized in both civil and criminal proceedings (Stuart, 2003b).

In light of the cottage industry that has grown up around identifying and managing dangerousness, mental health professionals lack credibility in leading anti-stigma programs designed to remove common stereotypes such as those dealing with violence and unpredictability. Yet mental health professionals are adept at this type of double-messaging. For example, in their review, Powell and Lloyd (2001) recommended that the following measures be implemented to insure the safety of community mental-health researchers in Exeter, England, who were required to complete face-to-face interviews with mental health clients in a variety of community settings. They were advised to negotiate contracts that acknowledged that it might not be possible to: interview as many users as planned if the researcher had a safety concern; incorporate additional costs into the contract in case researchers needed to be escorted to an interview; arrange interviews in non-domiciliary environments; end an interview if a researcher felt at risk; advise interviewers not to carry visible valuables such as a laptop computer; arrange interviews prior to dusk; and have emergency systems in place if an interviewer did not report back to the base by a specified time. Some of these recommendations, such as making sure that emergency systems were in place, would be sage advice for any study group, whether or not people with a mental illness were involved. However, keeping laptops out of sight and renegotiating research contracts on the expectation that there will be significant safety concerns seem to reflect deeply held stereotypes and provide further examples of situations that undermine professionals' credibility with respect to anti-stigma messaging. In many Eastern European countries, psychiatrists had longer annual vacations because they claimed that they were dealing with dangerous people. Until recently, in the United Kingdom, earlier retirement from service could be requested on the same grounds.

Finally, the possibility of coercive practices in mental-health care has a chilling effect on the credibility of mental health professionals assuming the leadership role in anti-stigma activities. Fear of coerced treatment has been identified as a significant barrier to help-seeking for people with a mental illness. Having been involuntarily detained in a mental hospital or general psychiatric unit is not only fraught with vocational, social, and legal repercussions, it is also a highly stigmatizing event (Arboleda-Flórez, 2011). Even when treatment is voluntary, there is often a veiled threat or coercive persuasion. In one study of mandated care in Northern California (Swartz, Swanson, and Hannon, 2003), 104 people with schizophrenia spectrum disorders and 85 mental health professionals were surveyed. The majority of the clinicians (78%) reported that they thought legal pressures made their patients more likely to stay in treatment, and 81% disagreed that mandated community treatment would deter a voluntary patient from seeking treatment in the future. Over a third of the patients (36%) reported that fear of coerced treatment was a barrier to help-seeking, particularly among the 63% who had previously experienced mandated care. Reminders or warnings about the consequences of treatment non-adherence were experienced as coercive and were also considered to be a barrier to care. As well as having a negative effect on treatment-seeking, the possibility of coercive practices in mental health care systems also undermines trust.

WHAT CAN MENTAL HEALTH PROFESSIONALS DO DIFFERENTLY?

The need to fight stigma and discrimination has been recognized by a number of professional bodies involved in the delivery of mental health care. In the last two decades, many—such as the World Psychiatric Association (Sartorius and Schulze, 2005) or the Royal College of Psychiatrists in the United Kingdom (Crisp, 2000)—have initiated anti-stigma programs. This is a departure from the usual situation where anti-stigma efforts are undertaken almost exclusively by community advocacy groups composed of people with lived experience of a mental illness.

Schulze (2007) has noted that, despite some noteworthy successes, anti-stigma programs originating from inside the profession have often been veiled attempts to raise the profile of psychiatry (or other mental health profession) rather than serious attempts to improve the situation of people who live with a mental illness. Official goals of professional programs have been openly challenged as little more than efforts to increase the use of mental health services and strengthen dependency on professional "fixes." Finally, professionals have been criticized for having focused on everyone else's attitudes but their own.

The knowledge that stigma is a major barrier to recovery imposes a clear duty on all health professionals and health systems to act. Perhaps, the first thing that psychiatrists and mental health professionals can do to reduce stigma is recognize that they are a key part of the problem. Secondly, it is important to recognize that it is possible to go beyond being part of the problem to being part of the solution. This requires a willingness to examine personal attitudes and behaviors with the goal of increasing one's tolerance and capacity to provide effective and humane care. Continuing to update one's knowledge about mental illnesses and listening to what patients and their families have to say about stigma and its consequences would greatly assist both of these tasks (Sartorius, 1998). Often it is the little thing that makes the most difference: a police officer who got an emergency room client a cup of coffee; a nurse who stayed beyond her shift to complete a conversation; a doctor who looked in her patient's eyes instead of in the chart when asking questions; or a pat on the arm with a kind word for a person on an emergency stretcher.

Careless use of diagnostic labels by health and mental health professionals is an important source of stigma. While diagnoses are useful tools in medicine when summarizing information about a patient's illness, they can be harmful if used in cavalier ways. Becoming more conscious of the stigmatizing power of a diagnosis and the psychological effects of the labeling process would contribute to a wiser and more careful use of diagnostic labels. Remembering that people are not their diagnoses—that they are people who are facing a mental health challenge—also would be helpful. Psychiatrists and mental health personnel must become aware that prognostic nihilism, use of terminology such as *schizophrenic* or *chronic*, suggestions that an individual must lower their expectations, or actions that exclude an individual from decision-making can be personally devastating. People with a mental illness need to be actively involved in their treatment and make full and informed decisions about treatment options.

When conducting research to measure personal experiences with stigma and discrimination (Stuart, Milev, and Koller, 2005), we were surprised to find out how much people wanted to talk about their stigma experiences. They provided extensive, rich accounts in response to open-ended questions, sometimes following up with detailed email descriptions of encounters. They often thanked the researchers for listening and were appreciative that someone was finally asking them about something that had come to take such a looming role in their lives. In recruiting clinic patients for this research, researchers were rarely if ever declined—a much different experience from the challenges faced when recruiting patients for other studies such as randomized drug trials. Therapists who assisted in collecting data using the study instruments often remarked at how much they had learned about the difficulties their patients were experiencing—which they had known little or nothing about. Though these instruments were developed for research purposes, their open-ended format provided a useful tool for the therapists to initiate discussions with both clients and family members. This has led to our belief that the topics of stigma, self-stigma, stigma management, and disclosure strategies should become regular components of the therapeutic encounter (see appendix for instruments).

Many psychotropic medications cause visible side-effects that are highly stigmatizing. Apart from side-effects that affect libido and one's relational life with a partner, extrapyramidal signs or weight gain, for example, may mark the person as having a mental illness and may be experienced as profoundly disturbing and painful. Obesity related to antipsychotic medications can erode one's self-esteem and interfere with one's ability to interact socially, in addition to increasing the risk of cardiovascular and other chronic diseases. Health care organizations and insurance plans will often support the use of cheaper medications, even when they are associated with disturbing side-effects; and consider medications with fewer side-effects to be too costly to be included in drug formularies. Medical practitioners tend to accept these policies without considering the importance of fighting to make sure that their patients have access to the best available treatments, even when they are not the cheapest. Being reluctant to pay for more expensive and more effective treatment for people with a mental illness clearly indicates decision makers' stigmatizing opinions—that mental illnesses are incurable and people with a mental illness are valueless, such that costlier medications would be wasted if given to them (Sartorius, 2002b).

At the system level, mental health professionals can be strong advocates for equitable treatment for people with a mental illness, both within health systems and at the broader societal level. Those in teaching roles can help students learn about the importance of appropriate professional and political activism and promote the recognition that recovery means more than symptom control and disease management. Lending support to local anti-stigma initiatives, as partners, learning from others about the ways in which they have successfully battled stigma, and making this a regular topic of clinical, administrative, scientific, and policy exchanges would go a long way toward reducing stigmatization and increasing professional credibility in this sphere (Sartorius, 1998).

The current biomedically oriented education model does not effectively promote positive attitudes toward people with a mental illness and may entrench negative attitudes and therapeutic nihilism. An approach that focuses on prospects for recovery and the importance of learning positive and respectful ways of dealing with people who have a mental illness and their family members is required. Research has demonstrated that mental health professionals can be retrained to work collaboratively with their clients. For example, the Schizophrenia Fellowship of Victoria (Australia) worked with family service providers and a large public psychiatric service to provide training opportunities for staff. Their educational strategy emphasized the importance of creating opportunities for family caregivers to participate in the treatment process. A brief program, composed of two three-hour sessions, and an extended program of twelve weekly three-hour sessions were offered. Staff members who attended the extended training session demonstrated more positive pro-family attitudes and increased their contacts with family members. Similar attitude and behavioral change was not evident among those who attended the brief training session (Farhall, Webster, Hocking, Leggatt, Riess, and Young, 1998).

In considering what psychiatric professionals can do differently, Byrne (2000) has challenged them to consider a number of important questions, such as: "Could you give a talk on stigma next week?" "What have you done to reduce stigma?" "Is stigma in the teaching curriculum at your university?" "Do students receive formal teaching about stigma?" He notes that none of the standard British textbooks in psychiatry cite *stigma* in their indices; there is a dearth of social-psychiatric research on stigma; and there seems to be considerable personal resistance to engaging in stigma-reduction activities.

In this chapter, we have demonstrated that health and mental health professionals are worthy targets of stigma-reduction efforts and that their affiliation with a system that promotes the identification and management of dangerousness, and uses coercive treatment approaches, considerably undermines any credibility they may have as leaders of community-based anti-stigma programs. Professional training does not equip health or mental health professionals to lead anti-stigma efforts, and more likely, it entrenches stigmatizing attitudes and behaviors. Nevertheless, professionals can (and should) contribute to anti-stigma efforts: first by examining their own attitudes and behaviors, and second by partnering with local anti-stigma initiatives.

7

Paradigm 6: Improved Knowledge About Mental Illness Will Eradicate Stigma

THE NATURE OF PREJUDICE

No corner of the world is free from group scorn. Being fettered to our respective cultures, we ... are bundles of prejudice

—ALLPORT, *2000, p. 20*

There is an important distinction to be made between *prejudice* and *misconception*. Both are prejudgements, but a misconception is a prejudgement that is based on wrong information—an erroneous belief that can be relatively easily corrected with new knowledge. A prejudice, on the other hand, is an emotional antipathy toward something or someone that is rooted in a false and inflexible generalization that is highly resistant to change. Whereas it is possible to discuss misconceptions and rectify them with new knowledge, this is not the case with prejudice. People become highly emotional and resistant when their prejudices are confronted, and they will actively discount any information that challenges them (Allport, 2000).

One of the best illustrations of the backlash that can occur when mental health–related prejudices are directly confronted comes from one of the earliest attempts to educate the public about mental illnesses. Although many years have passed since this social experiment was conducted, it continues to stand out as one of the most critically reflective efforts to understand what went wrong. *Closed Ranks* (1957) documented the Cummings' attempts to reduce feelings of social distance toward people with a mental illness and improve the community's sense of social responsibility. It occurred at the end of the asylum era in a small Canadian prairie town; dubbed with the pseudonym "Blackfoot."

The Cummings based their anti-stigma activities on the assumption that ignorance and fear would be widespread among Blackfoot residents. Because they were likely to be dealing with relatively immovable ideas, they considered that it was unlikely that a traditional public-educational program using mass media messages would be particularly effective. They were aware that previous attempts to break down ethnic prejudices using such methods had proved disappointing. Therefore, they opted for a plan that was more tailored, intensive, and fluid—a good example of what we have described in Chapter 4 as "enlightened opportunism." The main thrusts of the educational program were to drive home three messages that (a) the causes of behavior are understandable and subject to change, (b) there is a continuum between normality and abnormality, and (c) there is a wider variety of "normal" behavior than people generally realize. Small group discussions led by people who were knowledgeable about mental health and mental illness were the preferred medium. However, the Cummings also capitalized on any opportunity that presented itself; for example, furnishing weekly articles for the local paper, broadcasting on a radio program, running school essay contests, and getting local groups to present a film festival. The most successful project was conducted by members of the Canadian Legion, who traveled 75 miles to visit veterans in the local mental hospital. The Legion members adopted one of the wards as a continuing project. They visited the patients and sent cigarettes, candies, and other comforts. After their first visit, they voted to include all of the patients, not just the veterans.

Over half of the population (56%) had some contact with the program during its six months of activity. Residents understood the intellectual content of the program, but had difficulty understanding the motivation. Initial reactions to the program were cordial, but as the program grew in momentum, so did the community's reactions. Within the first month, rumors began to spread. One was that the government had sent out the research team to investigate community attitudes toward mental illness because they were thinking about building a new mental hospital. A more nefarious rumor was that the program was a plot of the Roman Catholic Church, though this made little sense and its origin was unknown. Three months into the program, the Cummings noticed that residents were withdrawing from them, and this pattern grew increasingly familiar. Residents let the researchers know that they expected that the program's activities should soon wind down. Others spoke about the anxiety and hostility that the program had created. When the team arrived to conduct their second round of surveys, community members refused to be interviewed and withdrew from the investigation, indicating they were no longer interested. During the week of the re-survey, their reception grew increasingly cold and hostile, which culminated with the mayor asking the researchers leave town. The ranks had been closed. As one interviewer noted:

There were feelings of hostility coming through from people on the streets and in the restaurants and hotel; I felt we were being talked about. I felt a lot of anxiety floating around. ... I only met three or four people who looked upon the survey as useful (Cumming and Cumming, 1957, p. 42).

In their analysis of events, the Cummings realized that their assumptions about the nature of prejudice had badly missed the mark. A qualitative assessment of community residents' assumptions prior to implementing the program—if used as a basis for developing the program—would have been sufficient to highlight these problems and would have avoided the problem of "teaching" residents what they already knew. Evaluation data revealed that community residents perceived a much broader range of behavior as "normal" than did the professionals who were trying to teach them to be more tolerant of abnormality. The investigators were shocked at the respondents' denial of pathological conditions in the case histories that were read to them and their willingness to attribute even serious psychotic disorders to more understandable and acceptable social and environmental conditions (such as early childhood trauma). The community's definition of "true" mental illness was exceedingly narrow and largely restricted to those who had been hospitalized.

The researchers' second assumption—that behavior was understandable—was exactly the same assumption held by the Blackfoot population. The educators had assumed that the community would be ignorant about behavioral causes, but the causes of behavior that community members were "taught" through the educational program were in serious disagreement with the causes that they had worked out for themselves. Rather than clinical causes derived from psychiatric and psychological schools of thought, residents displayed a more concrete cause-and-effect logic that often linked bad experiences (especially in childhood) to adverse behaviors. For example, it seemed natural that, if one had been treated badly in the past, then one would have reason to feel persecuted in the present, so paranoid behavior had a "naturalness" about it. The program planning committee displayed considerable naïveté in their assumption that people needed professional advice to understand mental illnesses.

The program message that appeared to have caused the strongest emotional backlash was that there was a continuum between normality and abnormality, and that the dividing line was arbitrary and artificial. Rather than seeing the potential for a continuum, residents saw a sharp distinction between those who were mentally ill ("them") and those who were normal ("us"). Mental illness was seen as synonymous with behavior that was non-normative and unpredictable, whether or not it was clinically pathological. The element of unpredictability was a central and immutable diagnostic point in lay definitions of mental illness, which could not be reconciled with the notion of an illness continuum. Programmers had significantly underestimated the intensity of public prejudices and the immutability of stigmatizing views.

> *In short, it appeared from our interviews that the people of Blackfoot had fixed ideas about the causes of behaviour, both normal and deviant, about the proper way to treat the mentally ill, and about the correct amount of responsibility to assume in the matter. Our vigorous attempts to alter these important ideas were unsuccessful and resulted in our co-workers' virtual rejection from the community* (Cumming and Cumming, 1957, p. 110).

Twenty years later, D'Arcy returned to this small prairie community only to find that, despite the liberalization of views in many walks of Canadian life, including the development of the community mental health treatment philosophy, social distance toward those with a mental illness remained as entrenched as it ever was (D'Arcy, 1987).

CAN PREJUDICE RESPOND TO NUGGETS OF KNOWLEDGE?

In the era of evidence-based medicine, most clinical work must be rooted in a theoretical research base that explains why a given intervention is effective. In the anti-stigma world, most programs proceed without a research base, on the assumption that programmers know what needs to be done and can deliver interventions that work. Conventional practices for developing anti-stigma programs often pay little attention to the underlying theory; the causal chain of events that establishes what must be done to bring about change. Program planners operate with repertoires of established approaches, so program design often means working with some familiar "off-the-shelf" package without a close analysis of the match between the nature of the problem and the capacity of the intervention to bring about change (Rossi, Lipsey, and Freeman, 2004). As the Blackfoot experiment vividly demonstrated, programs may be based on faulty assumptions about the nature of prejudice and discrimination (Cumming and Cumming, 1957).

A common off-the-shelf solution for stigma-reduction programs is a large social-marketing campaign designed to increase awareness and improve public attitudes. The common *modus operandi* is to provide brief "nuggets of knowledge," such as: *One in five will experience mental illness in their lifetime*, or *Depression is treatable*. These are intended to demystify mental illnesses, explode myths, and normalize their occurrence. Such messaging is based on the assumption that providing people with improved knowledge of the facts will change their prejudices.

There is no supporting evidence from social psychology that knowledge can change deep-seated prejudices, particularly prejudices that are rooted in fear. In fact, the opposite seems to be true. People will selectively attend to information that supports their prejudices and actively ignore or discount information that contradicts them. Even in the face of considerable contradictory evidence, people can maintain their prejudices through a process of *re-fencing*. Contradictory evidence is not allowed to modify the prejudice, an exception is acknowledged, and the fence remains intact (Allport, 2000). A good example of the resilience of prejudice to information occurred in the 1970s acclaimed television sitcom titled *All in the Family*. The main character, Archie Bunker, was an ultra-conservative, reactionary, blue-collar bigot who, when his prejudices were confronted by his liberal son-in-law (dubbed "Meathead") would exclaim, "Don't confuse me with the facts!"

There is also a growing body of evidence to show that good mental health literacy coexists with high levels of social intolerance; so by changing one, you do not necessarily change the other. Two surveys from Canada illustrate this point. In 2007, the Canadian Alliance on Mental Illness and Mental Health showed that Canadians were relatively knowledgeable about mental illnesses and their treatments (Bourget and Chenier, 2007). The majority of respondents (79%) correctly identified depression from a vignette; almost half (45%) correctly identified schizophrenia; and over a third (39%) correctly identified anxiety. Respondents embraced a wide range of biomedical, social, and psychological causes, though they were more apt to link anxiety and depression to psychosocial causes and schizophrenia to biological ones. The majority recommended seeking medical help for symptoms of schizophrenia (66%), and depression (61%)—though less so for anxiety (46%).

In 2008, the Canadian Medical Association's annual national survey (Canadian Medical Association, 2008) reported that, when asked to pick between two alternate statements, nine in ten respondents (89%) said that mental illnesses were like cancer or diabetes in that they require treatment from a health professional. Only one in ten considered that mental illnesses did not require professional care. Seven in ten respondents agreed that funding for mental health services should be on par with funding for physical health issues, and six in ten agreed that mental health services were under-funded. However, when asked about the likelihood that they would interact socially with someone who had a mental illness or addiction, Canadians expressed high levels of social distance.

Only about half thought that they would socialize with a friend (58%) or colleague (49%) who had a mental illness. Less than a third (31%) would hire a landscaper, 15% a financial advisor, and 12% a lawyer with a mental illness. Only about one in ten (11%) would have a family doctor with a mental illness; 16% thought that they would enter a spousal relationship; and 14% thought that they would have someone with a mental illness take care of their children (Canadian Medical Association, 2008).

In addition, there is some evidence to show that improvements in mental health literacy do not correspond with decreases in negative or prejudicial attitudes. In the United States, for example, Phelan and colleagues compared public attitudes in 1950 and 1996 (Phelan, Link, Stueve, and Pescosolido, 2000). Public conceptions of mental illness had broadened significantly during that time to include a greater proportion of non-psychotic disorders, which more closely approached professional definitions. At the same time, stereotypes of violence and other frightening characteristics linked to mental illnesses increased. For example, in 1950, 7% of respondents mentioned violent incidents or manifestations in relation to mental illnesses, compared to 12% in 1996. Among those who equated mental illnesses with psychosis, mentions of manifestations of violence increased from 13% in 1950 to 31% in 1996.

Also in the United States, Pescosolido and colleagues (Pescosolido, Martin, Long, Medina, and Link, 2010) examined changes in knowledge about the causes of mental illnesses and public stereotypes between 1996 and 2006. In 2006, a greater proportion of the public embraced neurobiological explanations for schizophrenia, depression, and alcohol-dependence. Public endorsement for medical treatments also increased. Eighty-five percent recommended that the person portrayed in the depression vignette should go to a psychiatrist (up from 75% in 1996), and 79% recommended specialty treatment for alcohol dependence (up from 61% in 1996). There was also a significant increase in the proportion of respondents who endorsed the prescription of medications. Despite this improved knowledge, there was no corresponding decrease in any indicator of public stigma, and levels of intolerance remained high. The majority of respondents continued to express social distance, such as an unwillingness to work or socialize with the person depicted in the vignette, and attributions of violence and dangerousness were unchanged. Of particular interest was the fact that neurobiological conceptions were either unrelated to stigma or actually increased the odds of a stigmatizing reaction.

Two representative surveys conducted in the eastern part of Germany in 1993 and 2001 showed similar results (Angermeyer, Holzinger, and Matschinger, 2009). In 2001, the percentage of respondents correctly identifying schizophrenia and depression from a vignette increased. Biological etiologies and professional treatments (such as psychotropic medication and psychotherapy) were also more highly endorsed. But the public's desire for social distance from people with either schizophrenia or depression remained largely unchanged. The authors concluded that these results do not support the assumption underlying many anti-stigma programs that improved attitudes will result from increased knowledge.

WHAT ABOUT MENTAL HEALTH LITERACY?

Considering that many programs target knowledge to improve mental health literacy, it is important to assess the concept of *mental health literacy* and examine the consequences of improved literacy for stigma reduction. Jorm (2000), who introduced the term, defines mental health literacy as the knowledge and beliefs about mental illnesses that promote their prevention, recognition, and management. In addition to recognizing specific symptoms, one must also know: when they are indicative of a mental disorder or significant psychological distress; that treatments are available; and where to access them. As well as encompassing knowledge and beliefs about what treatments are available, mental health literacy includes attitudes that promote recognition and help-seeking. Information campaigns that target public awareness about the frequency, symptoms, or treatment options for a particular mental illness are an example of a program based on literacy theory. For literacy-based programs, the ultimate (distal) endpoint is the reduction of disability through improved recognition and help-seeking. For anti-stigma programs, the ultimate endpoint is the reduction of social discrimination. One is based on a medical model; the other on a human rights and social justice model.

Research has shown that simple literacy messages of the type that could be used in population-based campaigns can improve attitudes toward treatment, but they may be insufficient to change the burden of disability (Gabriel and Violato, 2010). For example, in Australia, Jorm and colleagues (Jorm, Griffiths, Christensen, Korten, Parslow, and Rodgers, 2003) compared an evidence-based consumer guide describing treatment for depression with a general brochure on depression. Subjects were drawn from a representative community sample. If they screened positive for depressive symptoms, they were randomly assigned to receive one of the interventions. The study found some changes in beliefs about treatment and actions such as trying a self-help treatment or giving advice to another, but no significant effect on professional help–seeking, symptoms, or disability. The authors suggested that evidence-based consumer guides are unlikely to have much effect unless used as a complement to other, more active, interventions.

Subsequently, Jorm and colleagues (Jorm, Christensen, and Griffiths, 2005) evaluated whether a population-based literacy campaign, *Beyondblue: The National Depression Initiative*, increased the Australian public's ability to recognize depression or influenced their beliefs about treatment. Using data from two national surveys (one completed in 1995 and one in 2004), researchers showed that recognition of depression from a case vignette increased in both the states that had high and low exposure to the *Beyondblue* messaging. In 2004, two-thirds of the sample correctly recognized depression, reflecting a 25% to 30% improvement over the previous survey. In addition, ratings of the likely helpfulness of different treatment interventions also improved over the eight-year period for most interventions, with greater improvements in the areas having high exposure to *Beyondblue*, suggesting that the literacy campaign had been successful.

Some mental health literacy programs have increased stigma. For example, Griffiths et al. (2004) randomly assigned 165 people to a depression-literacy website and 182 to a cognitive-therapy-therapy skills training site. The depression website provided information about symptoms of depression, sources of help, evidence-based information about interventions, and information about the prevention of depressive disorders. It also included short biographies of famous people who had experienced depression. The cognitive-therapy intervention provided methods for overcoming dysfunctional thinking, and facilitating relaxation, problem-solving, assertiveness training, and other self-help strategies. Each module directed participants to read more about depression and its treatment. Both interventions resulted in small but statistically significant drops in negative attitudes relative to the control group. However, those in the cognitive-behavioral training intervention showed an increase in extent to which they thought *others* stigmatized people with a mental illness. The authors speculated that the emphasis on changing thoughts and behaviors in the cognitive-behavioral model may have led participants to believe that others view depression as controllable. They also considered that mental health literacy programs that emphasize improved understanding of the illness and illness-management may be sub-optimal for addressing stigma, and suggested that approaches that focused directly on stigma reduction would be required.

Mental Health First Aid courses have gained popularity as a means of improving mental health literacy. Originally developed in Australia by Kitchener and Jorm (2002) they have since been applied widely to various target groups— often members of the general public who will have frontline contact with people who have a mental illness. The nine-hour course is intended to provide basic skills to allow someone to help in a mental health crisis by (a) assessing risk of suicide or self-harm, (b) listening in a non-judgemental manner, (c) giving reassurance and information, (d) encouraging the person to get appropriate professional help, and (e) encouraging self-help strategies. The training has been evaluated in both quasi-experimental and experimental studies and found to produce greater recognition of disorders, improved agreement with mental health professionals concerning which interventions are likely to be helpful, increased confidence in providing help for others, and increased help actually provided. In addition, some studies have found statistically significant reductions in social distance, though the magnitude of the change is small—on the order of 3% of the scale scores (Kitchener and Jorm, 2002).

When the Mental Health First Aid course was offered to staff in the Student Affairs Division at Queen's University in Canada (Massey, Brooks, Burrow, and Sutherland, 2010), no improvement in social distance was noted. Student affairs staff have frontline contact with students through the residences, hospitality services, career services, the International Center, health and disability counseling services, athletics, recreation, and a center for mature female students. An evaluation based on 84 participants showed that the training accomplished its key objectives of increasing knowledge and raising confidence. Compared to the untrained comparison group, the trained group scored significantly higher on the post-test knowledge scale (reflecting a large standardized effect size of 1.06). This reflected an increase of between 18% and 32% on every knowledge item. The largest increase in knowledge was for violence or aggressive behavior associated with mental health issues. Trained staff also reported increased knowledge of the wide range of mental health conditions, as well as improved knowledge pertaining to more serious illnesses.

With respect to recognition of people with a mental health condition, the trained group reported greater confidence in recognizing people with a mental health condition, and so reported greater contact with individuals with mental health problems in their day-to-day activities, as respondents were more able to identify individual's problems as mental health–related. The program significantly increased the staff's confidence in their ability to help someone and increased the likelihood of their engaging in helping, reflecting a large standardized effect size (1.28). The proportion of those who rated themselves as "confident" or "very confident" rose from 38% to 68%. Respondents who received the training were also more likely to assist in situations in which mental health was an issue. However, staff did not report greater openness to dealing with people who had a mental health condition (measured in terms of social distance). Interview data revealed that respondents—though more comfortable in interacting with people with mental health problems in the course of their daily activities—were still reticent about becoming socially involved with them, particularly if the illness were serious. People were willing to engage with people if they were in need of help, but would not go out of their way to spend time with them, or take the first step toward developing a social relationship. For example, one respondent stated: "If they needed me, I would be there in a heartbeat, but only long enough to make sure they were situated" (Massey, Brooks, Burrow, and Sutherland, 2010, p. 18). Other respondents indicated that they would not like to have someone with a mental illness marry into their family because it might place subsequent generations at risk through genetic transmission. These results illustrate that Mental Health First Aid was highly successful in meeting its literacy and first-aid goals, but did not improve the staff's willingness or desire to develop and maintain close social contacts with people who have a mental illness; however, these outcomes were not considered to be the main objectives of the program.

ANTI-STIGMA PROGRAMS AS PURVEYORS OF MEDICAL KNOWLEDGE

A mental health literacy perspective on stigma reduction often views lay conceptions as deficient approximations of professional beliefs. Anti-stigma programmers who adopt this perspective see their role as purveyors of medical knowledge to people who hold "incorrect" explanations for mental illnesses.

Lay people tend to use non-medical criteria to determine whether or not a person is mentally "abnormal" or has a mental "illness." This was first vividly highlighted in the Blackfoot study in Canada (Cumming and Cumming, 1957). Rather than using clinical models, Blackfoot residents used normative and moral frameworks that made it possible for them to reject ex-patients who had been cured of gross psychological symptoms as "as bad as ever" while accepting those who were still hallucinating or delusional as "cured." As the researchers learned, their attempts to change or replace normative frameworks with psychological ones resulted in resistance and hostility. As discussed in Chapter 3, in cultures that do not have a well-developed concept of mental illness, stigma is reserved for the behaviors and symptoms that grossly threaten the equanimity of the social group. A wide range of abnormal behaviors is deemed to be acceptable and understandable, particularly if they are considered to be the result of external, supernatural causes.

The qualities that lay people use to differentiate abnormal psychological symptoms from ones that are "normal" or "acceptable" have profound practical importance for understanding stigma and for stigma-reduction programs. Haslam (2005) has outlined a model of folk psychiatry with four dimensions that lay people use to conceptualize and stigmatize mental illnesses:

- Pathologizing—a judgment that a behavior is a gross deviation from some desirable standard;
- Moralizing—a judgment that the individual is morally accountable for their abnormality;

- Medicalizing—a judgment that the abnormality has a somatic basis; and
- Psychologizing—ascribing abnormality to psychological or emotional dysfunction.

The folk model predicts that medicalizing mental illnesses will foster negative attitudes both in the individual who has the illness, by promoting pessimism and self-stigma, and in the lay public, by stoking fears of immutability, unpredictability, distancing, and rejection. Attributing symptoms and behaviors to uncontrollable causes, such as chemical abnormalities, creates the perception that mentally ill individuals are unaccountable, irresponsible, and unpredictable. In addition, medicalizing encourages essentialist thinking that the "mentally ill" individual is deeply and categorically different from oneself. As discussed earlier in this chapter, there is growing evidence to show that lay explanations for mental illnesses are converging with professional biological definitions, without corresponding increases in social tolerance (Phelan, Link, Stueve, and Pescosolido, 2000): and in some cases, the "professional world view" corresponds to higher levels of stigma (Pescosolido, Martin, Long, Medina, and Link, 2010). Thus, when normative explanations for mental illnesses are supplanted by medical ones, stigma and social rejection may be increased.

There are differences between misconceptions that respond to information, and prejudices that are deep-seated and resistant to change. It is important to maintain a clear distinction between programs that are designed to reduce disability by improving mental health literacy and help-seeking, from those designed to decrease stigma and social rejection. There is a danger that increased understanding of the neurobiological basis for mental illnesses engenders stigma by sharpening divisions between what is considered "normal" and "abnormal" and by consolidating stereotypes of immutability, uncontrollability, and dangerousness.

8

Paradigm 7: Attitude Change Is
the Yardstick of Success

Targeting attitude change in the context of anti-stigma programming raises three thorny issues. The first is that attitudes are poor predictors of behaviors. The knowledge-attitude-behavior continuum that is at the root of much programmatic thinking in this field has not been well supported by empirical literature. The second difficulty concerns the fact that the evidence base supporting our ability to change attitudes is weak. Finally, if we are willing to overlook the problems that prejudicial attitudes do not correlate with behaviors, or that we do not have generalizable knowledge about how to influence them anyway, then we must face the fact that our best efforts to date have resulted in small and potentially irrelevant amounts of improvement.

THE KNOWLEDGE-ATTITUDE-BEHAVIOR CONTINUUM

All programs have a theory of change. Some are explicit, logical, and evidence-informed. Others (perhaps most) are not. These are poorly articulated, illogical, or inconsistent with best practices. Many anti-stigma programs are built on the logic of a three-step model. This model assumes that knowledge, attitudes, and behaviors lie along a continuum; and that to change behavior, one must first prepare the ground by changing knowledge (sometimes termed *awareness*) and then attitudes (see Figure 8.1). For example, the *See Me* Scottish campaign describes their program as informed by a model of a "journey" through a "virtuous cycle" that moves people through discrete steps that coalesce around the three dimensions of awareness raising, attitude change, and behavior change (Myers et al., 2009). Other campaigns and programs have not been so explicit, but their focus on correcting stereotypical content and attitude change suggests

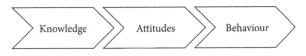

Figure 8.1 The three-step model of change.

that the knowledge-attitude-behavior continuum is also their underlying pro-gram theory.

The belief that prejudicial attitudes and discriminatory behaviors are closely related has not been borne out in the empirical literature. Indeed, prejudice has been a generally poor predictor of discrimination. Research shows that discrimination can occur in the absence of prejudice, and prejudice can occur in the absence of discrimination. For example, in a meta-analytic review of 60 studies published between 1930 and 1993, Schütz and Six (1996) concluded that prejudice was *only rarely* a valid predictor for discrimination. Only about 10% of the variation in measures of discriminatory behavior could be accounted for by variations in prejudicial attitudes. In addition, the strength of the relationship between prejudice and discrimination, though never strong, varied by measurement approach, target group, assessment strategies, and the time between measurements (with longer intervals yielding stronger correlations).

Figure 8.2 shows a more complex interplay between mental health literacy, prejudice, and discrimination. It shows a partial overlap between prejudice and discrimination and a paradoxical relationship between these and mental health literacy. In Chapter 11, we provide more detail on how improved knowledge, particularly about the neurobiological basis of mental illnesses, can improve attitudes, but at the same time increase public intolerance and desire for social distance. For our present purposes, it is sufficient to recognize that literacy-based programs that aim to improve knowledge about mental illnesses may not have the desired effect on discriminatory behaviors.

WHAT WE DON'T KNOW ABOUT PREJUDICE REDUCTION

Prejudices are fixed and largely immovable. This raises the important question of whether we have adequate empirical evidence to conclude that we know how to change prejudicial attitudes. Critics point to a lack of valid data, owing in part to a general lack of intervention research, the poor quality of study designs, and measurement complexities that make it difficult to interpret the meaning of changes.

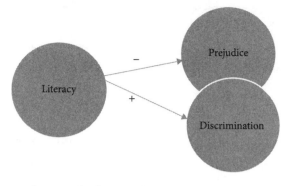

Figure 8.2 The complex interplay between literacy, prejudice, and discrimination.

Many of the most important theories about prejudice have grown out of public-opinion research designed to diagnose the origins of prejudice, largely in relation to racial prejudice. Rarely have interventions to ameliorate it been proposed or tested. Paluck and Green (2009) describe the theoretical and methodological sophistication of the prejudice literature as undeniable, but suggest that it has generated little valid practical knowledge that could be used in the field. In addition to the poor methodological quality of many studies, entire genres of prejudice-reduction interventions, which have now become commonplace (including diversity training, many educational programs, and sensitivity training), have never been evaluated using experimental field methods. Prejudice-reduction theories that have received the strongest support in laboratory studies have received little attention in the field. Consequently, it is necessary to extrapolate far beyond the existing evidence in order to formulate prejudice-reduction strategies.

Scholarly and scientific interest in mental illness–related stigma reduction is growing, though the evidence base needed to support best practices in the field is still meager and incommensurate with the burden of disability caused by stigma. In most countries, the funding that is made available to support mental health services research and evaluation is deficient. Consequently, few anti-stigma programs have been rigorously evaluated. A number of promising practices have been identified, but they have not been implemented widely enough to assess their impact on attitude change at a population level, their sustainability over time, their cost-effectiveness, or the extent to which attitude changes predict important behavioral outcomes. As is characteristic with the more general prejudice-reduction literature, systematic attempts to bridge laboratory-based experiments to real-world intervention programs do not exist on a large enough scale to inform public health practices (Stuart, 2009).

A further complicating factor is that expressed attitudes, elicited when respondents are directly asked what they believe, may be highly susceptible to reporting bias. In countries based on egalitarian philosophies, expressions of prejudice and discrimination are strongly discouraged. Thus, survey questions that are designed to elicit direct personal expressions of prejudice can generate socially desirable response sets, which occur when respondents give a more socially acceptable answer or deliberately mask their true feelings (Streiner and Norman, 1995).

In their studies in the United States, Link and Cullen (1983) have demonstrated that attitudinal responses toward people who have a mental illness are expressed at different levels. At the broadest level, respondents provide answers that are consistent with dominant ideological themes reflecting the most socially appropriate response. When asked directly about what they think or what they would do, their responses reflect an ideology of acceptance, or a social desirability response set. These overt expressions may bear little resemblance to more deeply held attitudes and are at odds with the day-to-day experiences of those who are victims of stigma. Thus, direct expressions of stigma not only underestimate the true level of rejection experienced by people with a mental illness, they are also problematic for assessing change over time. As anti-stigma messages become more forceful, it will be impossible to tell whether programs reflect true changes in prejudicial attitudes, or greater knowledge on the part of respondents concerning what constitutes a socially acceptable response. In this situation, not only will direct expressions of prejudice bear little relationship to behaviors and the lived experiences of people with a mental illness, they are likely to give highly misleading results about the effects of anti-stigma efforts.

Link and colleagues have suggested that more deeply held attitudes can be tapped by asking indirect questions, such as asking respondents how they think *most people* would respond to a particular statement. Indirect questions tap broad cultural predispositions, not the respondent's own personal attitudes and beliefs. The respondents can answer truthfully about ambient levels of prejudice without implicating themselves as stigmatizers, or revealing their own deeply held attitudes and beliefs (Link and Cullen, 1983). Such indirect measures are useful benchmarks for anti-stigma programming only when the target of the program is broadbased cultural-level change, such as in the case of a national campaign. For smaller, targeted programs, indirect measures will be insensitive to change because they do not measure the attitudes of the people who are receiving the intervention.

HOW MUCH CHANGE IS CHANGE?

One of the key challenges in any evaluation is determining the magnitude of change that will be required in order to declare an intervention successful. This information is also essential to obtain in order to adequately plan the sample size for the evaluation so that there are sufficient subjects to detect a statistically significant difference, if one exists. Small changes require large sample sizes, but large sample sizes have the disadvantage of having the power to detect statistically significant, yet practically meaningless, differences. Thus, having a clear idea of how much change is change is a key challenge for anti-stigma programmers and evaluators.

Program advocates typically proclaim lofty goals, expect unreasonably large effects, or believe in the possibility of program accomplishments that go beyond the program's ability to change (Rossi, Lipsey, and Freeman, 2004). Agreeing on performance standards is one of the most challenging aspects of anti-stigma programming. If changes are small and expectations are big, program participants may become discouraged and begin to transmit the message that stigma cannot be beaten. Choosing reasonable goals and managing expectations, both within the program and in the wider community, are central to the success of anti-stigma efforts. Setting aside the issue that attitudinal change may not give rise to changes in behaviors, the question of how much change is enough needs to be addressed by programs that target this dimension of stigma. Research shows that the amount of change realized typically has been small.

The *Like Minds, Like Mine* anti-stigma campaign in New Zealand has been tracking attitude change over eight national surveys following spates of intensive media advertising (Wyllie and Mackinlay, 2007). Survey questions include a number of attitude items as well as several questions designed to assess respondents' willingness to interact with someone with a mental illness. Considering the percent of the sample in each survey that responded in a non-stigmatizing manner, the average absolute percentage change has been approximately 4% on the attitude items and 3% on the social interaction (social distance) items. It is also important to note that not all of the item-level changes were in the desired direction.

Since March of 1993, the Department of Health in the United Kingdom has included stigma-related questions in their annual national Omnibus survey, which is designed to be representative of all adults in Great Britain. Data are available for 1994 to 2008, making it possible to assess changes in attitudes and desire for social distance over eight survey waves. Changes over time often have been small, with no obvious trend toward improvement. For example, agreement with the statement that "I would not want to live next door to someone who has been mentally ill" fluctuated between 8% and 13%, standing at 12% in 2008. A social-distance item that showed larger fluctuation but no real improvement reflected agreement that it was frightening to think that people with mental health problems were living in residential neighborhoods. In 1994, 15% agreed with this statement. This had increased to 26% in 1997, but settled back down to 16% in 2008.

These results illustrate that the average amount of change that could be expected in attitude and social distance measures from survey to survey is generally small (often less than 5%) and may fluctuate widely within items. Whether small attitudinal changes at the population level can give rise to meaningful improvements for people with a mental illness or their family members, or improve social inequities, is unknown, but unlikely. The Scottish *See Me* anti-stigma campaign is working from the assumption that it will take a generation to move through the knowledge-to-behavior continuum (Myers et al., 2009).

WHEN ARE ANTI-STIGMA PROGRAMS SUCCESSFUL?

When is an anti-stigma program successful? Rather than small improvements in public knowledge or attitudes, we would argue that an anti-stigma program can be considered to be successful only when (1) people who are stigmatized feel that their lives have been improved; (2) the impact of stigma on various life domains has been diminished; or (3) structures that promote inequity are removed or replaced with structures that protect and promote social entitlements in areas such as education, housing, health care, disability supports, training, or employment. The ultimate goal of anti-stigma programming, therefore, should not be knowledge or attitude change, but an improvement in areas of active participation and social inclusion, improved quality of life, and the fullest protections of social rights and entitlements.

Much of the existing stigma literature has focused on public expressions of stigma, and the yardstick for success has been change in public attitudes or behavioral intentions (as measured by social-distance scales). Given the potential for response bias, it is unlikely that small improvements in public attitudes signify meaningful changes in the day-to-day lives of people who have a mental illness, or of their family members. Furthermore, the link between attitude change and improved civic and human rights for people with a mental illness has not been demonstrated.

In 2007, after four years of intensive campaign activity by Scotland's *See Me* national campaign, people with a mental illness were surveyed to determine if they had experienced a reduction in stigma (McArthur and Dunion, 2007). Rather than using a population-based survey, respondents were recruited through promotions on the website and through community agencies. Three-quarters of the 1,100 volunteers reported experiencing a mental health problem in the previous five years, and the remainder had helped someone with a mental health problem. Nine out of ten could recall at least one of the campaign advertisements, and 63% considered that the *See Me* campaign had made a difference to how people with a mental illness viewed themselves. Fifty percent thought that there had been some or a little improvement in how others treat people with a mental health problem as a result of the campaign. Four percent thought there had been "a lot" of improvement, 10% thought there had been no improvement, and over a third (36%) were unsure. More than half (55%) reported noticing a change in the way the media reported stories about mental illness and their use of language; 25% noticed "a little" change, 23% "some" and 7% noticed "a lot" of change. The remainder (45%) reported no change. Although these results may be encouraging, they are not representative of all people with a mental illness, and they do not focus on changes in their own personal stigma experiences.

ENVIRONMENTS ARE NOT JUST CONTAINERS

Marshal McLuhan once said that "environments are not just containers, but are processes that change the content totally" (McLuhan, 1995, p. 275). So it is that an environment, through judicial, organizational, and other social structures, can create discrimination and inequity, even though people who are in it may not be prejudiced (at least at the outset). Through the process of socialization, environments have the ability to create a self-perpetuating cycle of stigma and discrimination, through multiple communication channels, making it difficult to unseat. Link and Phelan (2001) used the concept of "institutional racism" to sensitize us to the idea that considerable disadvantage can accrue to a group of individuals outside of the traditional anti-stigma model in which one person does something to another. The accumulated social and institutional practices that work to the disadvantage of minority groups can result in considerable discrimination even in the absence of personal prejudices. For example, disabled individuals may be limited in their ability to be socially included, not necessary because of any inherent limitation, but because they are in a disabling environment—one that erects barriers to their full and effective participation.

Disability discourse has shifted from a medical model that focuses on an individual's impairments and limitations, to a social and human rights model that focuses on the characteristics of society that make social participation impossible. From this perspective, stigmatization is viewed as a form of social oppression. In 2008, the United Nations Convention on the Rights of Persons with a Disability came into force to promote, protect, and ensure the full and equal enjoyment of human rights and fundamental freedoms for all people with a disability (including those with a mental or intellectual impairment; United Nations General Assembly, 2006). Under the convention, discrimination occurs when an impairment-related exclusion or restriction exists that impedes or nullifies the recognition, enjoyment, or exercise of human rights and fundamental freedoms on an equal basis with others. It includes all forms of discrimination: political, economic, social, cultural, and civic. Signatories to the convention (currently some 150 countries) agree to adopt sweeping social changes, including implementing appropriate legislative, administrative, and other reforms to ensure that the rights of people with physical or mental impairments are recognized. This has signaled an important shift in thinking about discrimination, from a model that emphasizes individual and interpersonal deficits, to one that highlights the importance of broad sociopolitical power structures and environmental factors.

In summary, focusing on attitude change as a consequence of anti-stigma programming is likely to yield disappointing results, both because the changes tend to be small and because attitude change is not a good predictor of behavioral change, which should be the main goal of anti-stigma programs. Therefore, it is unlikely that anti-stigma programs that solely target changes in attitudes will result in meaningful improvements in social inclusion and social equity for people who have a mental illness. Social structures are an important target for change, given that they have the ability to create inequities even in the absence of individual prejudices.

9

Paradigm 8: Community Care Is Destigmatizing

STIGMA AS A CONSEQUENCE OF INSTITUTIONALIZATION

Mental health policy and programming has been rife with popular and professional myths relating to the characteristics of people with a mental illness and their treatment needs. These myths have been fuelled by widespread ignorance of the etiology and nature of mental illnesses, ideological and administrative rivalries, legal and administrative structures that elevate dangerousness and unpredictability over the need for treatment or the ability to benefit from care, media distortions, and lack of population-based epidemiological data. Thus in mental health reform, the good intentions of one generation provide the fodder for the apologies of the next.

Figure 9.1 depicts three eras of stigma discourse corresponding to three of the most recent policy paradigms shaping mental health service delivery. In the first paradigm (roughly from the 1950s to the 1970s in North America and Western Europe), stigma was viewed as a consequence of institutionalization. Institutions in this period had long since passed their prime, many of them having become overcrowded, anti-therapeutic warehouses that perpetuated human rights abuses and coercive treatment; and in such institutions people with a mental illness were often imprisoned and neglected. Friern Hospital (also known as the Colney Hatch Lunatic Asylum), for example, which opened in the United Kingdom in 1851, was built for 1,000 patients, but by 1951, it housed 2,400. Recreational spaces were filled with beds, and, because of the limited number of staff, patients did not receive individual attention, but block treatment complete with a depersonalizing hospital uniform (Leff and Warner, 2006).

In the United States, between 1880 and 1940, the number of persons in state mental hospitals increased five times faster than the general population,

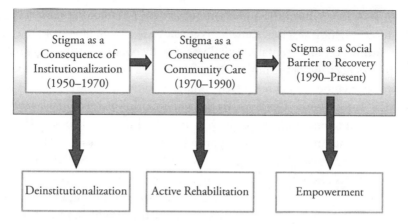

Figure 9.1 Stigma discourse.

reaching a peak of 445,000 residents. Most state hospitals lacked the basic resources needed to provide even minimal quality care. Legislature kept hospital operating budgets low. Physical plants became decrepit and overcrowded and it became increasingly difficult to attract and hold an adequate number of trained staff. Physical abuse of patients was a problem in many locations. By the 1950's the mentally ill occupied every other hospital bed in the country and scandalous exposés about the appalling conditions in these institutions were becoming more frequent. Many found expression in popular books, movies, and journalistic accounts. In addition to highlighting the deplorable conditions in institutions, they also helped to change the image of mental illness, by identifying the hospital itself, as a potential cause of disability—a conclusion that was reached by both the scholarly and the popular writers of the day (described in more detail below). In 1963, one month before President Kennedy's death, the Community Mental Health Centers act was signed into law, signaling the start of the community mental health movement (Rochefort, 1993).

In Canada, the asylum system expanded up until approximately 1960, when it reached its zenith of 66,000 inpatient beds. Most of the buildings dated from the Victorian era, with a patchwork of new construction to increase bed spaces and ease overcrowding. In 1932, Canadian asylums had 30% more patients than their rated bed capacity. Despite a doubling of beds between the 1930s and 1960s, in the 1960s they were still running at 10% over capacity, with some facilities housing as many as 5,000 individuals. Conditions were deplorable. By the 1950s, general hospital psychiatric units were just beginning to be developed (with only 11 in the entire country), and there were no treatment services or supports in the local community. The vocational and social rehabilitation needs of patients received virtually no attention, so that patients who were returned to their communities after hospitalization experienced considerable hardship. A report from the Royal Commission on Psychiatric Services, published in 1964, indicates that Canadians considered mental illnesses a deep disgrace. Admission to a mental hospital was usually obtained using legal means, with the cooperation of the police. Once admitted, a person all but disappeared, and family members quickly severed contact with them (Stuart, 2010).

In the early 1960s, Goffman published two seminal volumes analyzing the social experiences of people with a mental illness. Both emphasized the exclusionary nature of society's response to mental illnesses and the negative psychosocial impacts this had. In *Asylums: Essays on the Social Situation of Mental Patients and Other Inmates*, Goffman followed the social mortification that occurred as a consequence of institutionalization, noting the manner in which hospitals of the day stripped patients of their rights and relationships (Goffman, 1961). In *Stigma: Notes on the Management of Spoiled Identity*, Goffman described the process of self-mortification that occurred in response to stigma and discrimination (Goffman, 1963). Shortly following these publications, Scheff (1966) published his treatise on the effects of labeling, which gave further credence to the stigmatizing effects of institutionalization. Building on Goffman's work, a central tenet of Scheff's "Labeling Theory" was that it was the diagnostic label of a mental illness, created through contact with the mental health system of the day, and the resulting stigma (rather than the impairments themselves) that created and maintained the disability. A number of other influential works were published during this time that also raised serious questions about the therapeutic qualities of mental institutions and the ability of organized psychiatry to correctly diagnose and effectively treat mental illnesses. Among the most prominent were Laing's *Divided Self* (1965), Rosenhan's *On Being Sane in Insane Places* (1974), Foucault's *Madness and Civilization* (1975), and Szasz's two volumes: *The Myth of Mental Illness* (1974) and *Psychiatric Slavery* (1977). These challenged the foundations of the medical model and vilified psychiatric institutions. This process was echoed in popular media, such as Kesey's semi-autobiographical novel *One Flew Over the Cuckoo's Nest* (1962)—whose 1975 movie-version images still color public perceptions of hospitalization and treatment—as well as movies such as *The Snake Pit* and *Pressure Point* (Wedding, Boyd, and Niemiec, 2005).

In a relatively short span of time, mental institutions in industrialized countries had become the object of policy concern and the focus of structural reforms. In developing countries, particularly those with a colonial heritage, large mental hospitals were located at considerable distances from urban centers. They were the only institutions in which the bulk of psychiatrists worked. Traditional healers and some private practice psychiatrists were the only other sources where people with a mental illness could seek care, and this continues to be the situation in many countries today.

Mechanic and Rochefort (1990) describe an ideological consensus that emerged during the early 1960s that provided the political energy to move away from the "Dark Ages" of institutionalism toward a New Age based on scientific and humanitarian principles. In announcing the Community Health Centers Act of 1963, President John F. Kennedy set a quantifiable target for deinstitutionalization—a 50% reduction in the number of patients under custodial care over the next 10 to 20 years. By 1975, the number of patients had declined by 62% (from a peak of 559,000 in 1955), reflecting an exodus of much larger proportions than originally outlined by the policy targets. By 1985, despite the growing overall population, the institutional census had dropped further, to 110,000. The speed with which these targets were achieved revealed a rare degree of fervent enthusiasm amongst health professionals and advocates, public officials, and members of the general public.

Similar trends have been reported elsewhere, though the time frames vary. In Canada, for example, most provinces had begun dismantling public mental hospitals by 1960. Between 1960 and 1980, the number of inpatient beds dropped from 69,128 to 20,301, reflecting a 71% reduction. Psychiatric beds went from four beds per 1,000 to less than one bed per 1,000 (Sealy and Whitehead, 2004). In Queensland, Australia, the volume of patients admitted to psychiatric institutions remained relatively steady between 1900 and 1950, at 38 patients per 10,000. By about 2000, this had dropped to 0.8 patients per 10,000 (Doessel, Scheurer, Chant, and Whiteford, 2005). Shorter (2007) compared the number of beds in state psychiatric hospitals as a percentage of total psychiatric beds in the European states and candidate states between 1972 and 2001. There were a number of countries, such as Hungary, where the asylum never predominated. For most of the European Union states, however, the reverse has been true. The proportion of beds in psychiatric hospitals has rapidly declined, reflecting what Shorter termed a "massive political and cultural assault" on the very idea of mental hospital care—the most extreme example being Italy, where public mental hospitals were abolished by an act of parliament.

Despite these important (and large) reductions, the majority of European Union countries still support large state psychiatric structures and they remain the norm in many developing countries (see Table 9-1). According to the World Health Organization's atlas of mental health resources, most of the world's population still has little or no access to even the most basic mental health treatments. A third of the countries reporting to the WHO *Mental Health Atlas* project in 2005 had no specified budget for mental health programming, and one in five spent less than 1% of their total health budget on mental health (WHO, 2005). Two-thirds of the world's population had access to less than one psychiatric hospital bed per 10,000, and more than half of the beds remained in large custodial institutions (WHO, 2001). In some countries, the institutional

Table 9-1. STATE PSYCHIATRIC BEDS, EUROPEAN UNION.

Percentage of Total Beds in a State Psychiatric Hospital	European Union States and Candidate States as of 2001
Less than 30%	Denmark
	Finland
	Italy
	Portugal
	Hungary
30–59%	Greece
	Bulgaria
	Slovenia
	Sweden*
	United Kingdom*
60–80%	Belgium
	France
	Germany
	Luxembourg
	Estonia
	Poland
	Romania
	Slovakia
More than 80%	Austria
	Ireland
	Netherlands
	Spain
	Czech Republic
	Latvia
	Lithuania
	Malta

*Based on 1982 figures. (Adapted from Shorter, 2007, p. 24.)

custodians have long since forgotten the patients' names, so they use numbers to identify them.

Public opinion about psychiatric hospitals remains negative. The Victorian image of a psychiatric hospital remains—a large-scale and forbidding institution located on the outskirts of the community, with locked doors and a custodial mandate. Once admitted, patients seldom get out (Sartorius et al., 2010).

Based on the assumption that "large mental hospitals or asylums can easily contribute to stigma," the European Union Green Paper on mental health reform has called for further deinstitutionalization and the establishment of services in primary care, community care, and general hospitals as part of a larger strategy to destigmatize mental illnesses and promote social inclusion. It is expected that the provision of community-based alternatives will provide opportunities for social inclusion and a better quality of life for people with a mental illness (Health and Consumer Protection Directorate-General, 2005, p. 11). Repeatedly over the past 40 years, the World Health Organization has similarly called for mental health reforms that would increase community resources for mental health care worldwide and improve the provision of mental health treatment within primary care (WHO, 2001).

STIGMA AS A CONSEQUENCE OF COMMUNITY CARE

The earliest asylums were places of refuge and protection that were intended to be restorative, not the human warehouses they eventually came to be. By the early 1970s, the asylum era was coming to a close. In most industrialized countries, it was supplanted by a new romance with the concept of providing services and supports in the community, including inpatient hospitalization in general hospital psychiatric units. The philosophy of community psychiatry had advanced the idea that mental illnesses were related to social, institutional, and biological factors, rather than individual factors. In this era, people with a mental illness increasingly came to be seen as a group that deserved social and policy support, and this shift in perception led to the development of less socially isolating and, it was thought, less socially stigmatizing treatments (Rochefort, 1993). Opening the doors to the outside world greatly increased the contacts between people with a mental illness and the general public. Stigma, which had previously focused on the concept of madness and the psychiatric institution, now shifted to the people themselves, and negative stereotypes multiplied (Guimon, 1999).

Researchers who were interested in following the paths of deinstitutionalized patients after their discharge from the hospital soon noted a pattern of transinstitutionalization. Some went to nursing homes, but many more found their way into jails and prisons. Fazel and Danesh (2002) identified 62 surveys of prisoners from 12 industrialized countries that had been published between 1966 and 2001, reflecting data on over 23,000 prisoners. Countries surveyed included Australia, Canada, Denmark, Finland, Ireland, the Netherlands, New Zealand, Norway, Spain, Sweden, the United Kingdom, and the United States. Approximately one out of every seven prisoners met the criteria for a psychotic illness or major depression. One in two male prisoners and one in five female prisoners met the criteria for an antisocial personality disorder. Compared to the general population, this reflected a two- to fourfold excess in psychosis and major depression and a tenfold excess in antisocial personality disorder. Extrapolating these figures to the United States alone, Fazel and Danesh estimated that there were several hundred thousand prisoners that may have psychosis or depression—a total that was twice the number of patients in all American psychiatric hospitals combined. Given the limited mental health resources in most jails and prisons, most prisoners with a mental illness are not receiving appropriate care. They also pointed out that about two-thirds of the world's prisoners live in developing countries where prison conditions would be much worse. Thus, it would seem that the community-care era has taken us full circle to when people with mental illnesses were imprisoned and neglected.

In some countries, highly specialized forensic mental health systems have developed. However, the forensic label that is assigned to someone who has a mental illness and has committed (or allegedly committed) a criminal act triggers additional exclusionary processes, even within the mental health system. Forensic clients experience a double stigma, which more severely compromises their ability to access employment and housing opportunities. Even community mental health agencies tend to screen out forensic clients. They are viewed by the public as potentially more violent than the average service-user, and as a consequence, may be required to undergo extended periods of compulsory community treatment—periods that may exceed the length of any criminal sentence that could have been levied (Livingston, Rossiter, and Verdun-Jones, 2011).

Access to care while in the community has emerged as another important problem. In 2004, Kohn and colleagues reported on the extent of the worldwide treatment gap, using data from 37 published community-based epidemiological studies on service utilization. The median percent of those who received treatment for schizophrenia and non-affective psychoses was 32%; for major depression and dysthymia, 56%; for bipolar disorder, 50%; for panic disorder, 56%; for generalized anxiety disorder, 58%; and for obsessive compulsive disorder, 60%. Seventy-eight percent of people who met the criteria for alcohol abuse or dependence did not receive treatment, making this the area with the largest gap (Kohn, Saxena, Levav, and Saraceno, 2004). The World Health Organization's Mental Health Consortium Surveys (2005) reported that 35% to 50% of people with serious mental disorders who were living in the community in developed countries did not receive treatment in the year prior to the survey. In developing countries, this gap was as high as 76% to 85%. While there are both social and structural reasons for these gaps, research has also shown that many people choose not to pursue mental health treatments, even when they are available, in order to avoid being labeled and stigmatized (Ben-Zeev, Young, and Corrigan, 2010).

The shift from the hospital to community mental health care has highlighted the role of the general practitioner in the treatment of people with mental health and emotional problems—even serious illnesses such as schizophrenia—as a destigmatizing alternative to specialty care. In Australia, where there is universal access to health care, three-quarters of general practitioners are actively engaged in treating patients with schizophrenia. At any given time, the typical general practitioner is managing two patients with schizophrenia conjointly with other specialist services, and one without specialty support (Carr et al., 2004).

In most parts of the world, people with mental illnesses tend to have less access to primary care and may experience a lower quality of care for their physical health problems. Diagnostic overshadowing appears to be common, such that physical health problems are misattributed to mental illnesses. Higher than average rates of physical illnesses, such as cardiovascular disease, obesity, diabetes, and HIV/AIDS, coupled with inferior treatment, increases the risk of premature death (Thornicroft, Rose, and Kassam, 2007). A 2006 survey of primary-care physicians in seven countries (Australia, Canada, Germany, New Zealand, the Netherlands, the United Kingdom, and the United States) showed that 30% to 60% of practices were not prepared to provide optimal care for patients with mental health problems (Schoen, Osborn, Huynh, Doty, Peugh, and Zapert, 2006).

Family physicians and general practitioners also have been reported to be more stigmatizing than psychiatrists and mental health providers, and more pessimistic about prognosis and recovery. Considerable research has shown that doctors and nurses hold negative and pejorative stereotypes about people with a mental illness—stereotypes that are comparable to those held by people with little or no clinical education, such as health care assistants (Raistrick, Russell, Tober, and Tindale, 2008), hospital cleaning staff (Ayduin, Yigit, Inandi, and Kirpinar, 2003), or members of the lay public (Stuart and Arboleda-Flórez, 2001).

Stigmatizing views are widely held to result in treatment disparities for people who have a mental illness, though this explanation ignores important patient and environmental factors that may also lead to treatment inequities. In the United States, Druss and colleagues (2000) found that patients with a myocardial infarction and a comorbid mental illness were less likely to be admitted to hospitals with transluminal coronary angioplasty (PCTA) or open-heart surgical facilities, and less likely to be transferred to such a facility once admitted. Patients with a mental illness were significantly less likely to have a cardiac revascularization procedure, and there were deficiencies in the quality of care provided on five established indicators: reperfusion, aspirin, beta-blockers, angiotensin-converting enzyme inhibitors, and smoking-cessation counseling. Moreover, these differences accounted for a substantial portion of the excess mortality noted among patients with a mental illness (Druss, Bradford, Rosenheck, Radford, and Krumholz, 2001). Treatment disparities have also been reported in diabetic care (Frayne et al., 2005); management of HIV/AIDS (Himelhoch et al., 2007); preventative services such as screening for cancer, receipt of immunization, or tobacco counseling (Desai, Rosenheck, and Perlin, 2002); and asthma management (Baxter, Samnaliev, and Clark, 2009), though the presence or extent of treatment disparities varies by location and by diagnostic group, with some groups having greater-than-average access to care.

The extensive treatment gaps that have characterized the community mental health era can be traced back to an active process of stigmatization that operates overtly and covertly to create and maintain structural inequities that limit access to necessary treatments, community supports, and economic opportunities. The placement of patients into communities has not decreased the stigma of mental illness. Rather, the massive resettlement of deinstitutionalized patients into ill-prepared communities and community-treatment systems has exacerbated negative attitudes and contributed to the higher morbidity and mortality.

STIGMA AS A SOCIAL BARRIER TO RECOVERY

There is a growing recognition that modern community-based mental health reforms have been seriously undermined by public fear and intolerance and by health and mental health systems that have been experienced as disempowering, disrespectful, and punitive. In response, people with mental illnesses are increasingly challenging mental health providers to provide recovery-oriented care. In this context, *recovery-oriented care* goes beyond traditional notions of disease management, in which patients are educated about how to adhere to medication regimens and prevent relapses, to supports and services that are empowering and help people gain new meaning and purpose. Empowerment, self-acceptance, autonomy, collaboration with health professionals, hope, and destigmatization are among the central themes of the recovery movement (Liberman and Kopelowicz, 2005).

The recovery movement emerged in the 1960s and 1970s among people who had experienced mental health treatment, variously termed *consumers*, *survivors*, or *ex-patients*. It began with a desire for broad recognition of the social oppression they had experienced, which culminated in human-rights violations, marginalization, and discrimination. The recovery paradigm has increasingly gained acceptance over the last several decades, so much so that that few mental health services in industrialized countries would not now claim to be "recovery-oriented." But providing recovery-oriented care is much more than a simple claim of doing so. It means a massive shift in thinking, service orientation, and use of resources. Recovery-oriented care "recognizes the person's ultimate centrality to care and that the involvement of services in someone's life is a privilege and not an automatic rite of passage" (Glover, 2005, p. 2). It also aims to eradicate professional stigma of people with lived experience of a mental illness.

The recovery movement can be defined both systemically, in terms of the redistribution of professional power within the mental health system, and individually, in terms of taking control and responsibility for one's life. It also looks beyond health and mental health systems to social forces that discriminate against people with a mental illness. Stigma reduction is an application of recovery principles to the broader community. The recovery model differs dramatically from the active rehabilitation model that promoted social inclusion from a professional power base (Jacobson and Curtis, 2000).

There have been many negative consequences for people with a mental illness as a result of the rapid deinstitutionalization of mental hospitals without appropriate community services to provide a safety net. These have included criminalization, increased stigmatization, social exclusion, poor quality of care, and poorer health outcomes. These problems challenge the notion that the community mental health movement has been a destigmatizing force leading to greater social participation for people with a mental illness. Because they are now more visible, and often less supported by treatment systems, people with a mental illness living in the community may be at greater risk of experiencing social stigma.

10

Paradigm 9: Anti-stigma Campaigns Work

It is tempting, if the only tool you have is a hammer, to treat everything as if it were a nail

—MASLOW, *1966, p. 15.*

THE CAUSE DE JOUR

Major anti-stigma campaigns of limited duration—say two or three, or even five years—may bring more harm than good. People with mental illnesses and their families, who are often only peripherally engaged in such campaigns, feel let down once the campaign is over and public attention is drawn to another cause de jour. While well-focused campaigns may lead to a change in knowledge or attitudes, they are unlikely to alleviate some of the most disturbing consequences of stigma. Anti-stigma work should not be conducted as a campaign (signifying a time limited burst of activity), but should instead become a routine part of health and other social services. Meaningful changes—those that will remove social injustices faced by people living with a mental illness—will take more time and more focused action.

Anti-stigma campaigns are universal in perspective, meaning they target the entire public in order to bring about change at the population level. Because they must reach so many people, universal programs typically rely on media such as television or radio to get their messages across. Thus, they are often expensive, time-limited, and thin on content. Public service announcements (via television or radio) that are designed to educate the public about mental illnesses are an example of a typical population based strategy. In chapters 7 and 8, we demonstrated that small improvements in knowledge or attitudes (typical of population-based efforts) may have limited (or no) impact on entrenched social inequities. The prospects for some useful effect are better when media campaigns are part of a broader and long-lasting anti-stigma program because they can act as boosters to the program. Unfortunately, they are often the intervention of choice for national anti-stigma efforts.

Media campaigns face a number of important logistical issues that limit their reach. Even well-funded and well-crafted public service announcements may fail to make an impact because they do not reach the intended audiences. Announcements may be presented outside peak viewing hours; audiences generally fail to remember the ads; or prejudicial attitudes may block key messages. Public service announcements also have a short shelf life. Audiences become habituated to the messages and quickly begin to tune them out; radio or television producers move on to promote other causes; the celebrities that are often used to make public service announcements lose their appeal or, in some cases, place time limits on the use of their material; or messages are lost in the din of the many other social marketing appeals that regularly compete for peoples' attention. Funding for these campaigns is also time-limited, so finding new funding to create new announcements remains a significant and sometimes insurmountable challenge (Corrigan, Roe, and Tsang, 2011).

When evaluating potential avenues for stigma reduction, the Canadian pilot program for the World Psychiatric Association's *Open the Doors* global anti-stigma program undertook a population-based radio campaign to convey the message that schizophrenia was treatable. The radio spots used a local psychiatrist and several people who were living with schizophrenia to add an element of contact to the approach, as contact-based education had been identified as a promising practice in the field (Corrigan et al., 2001). The psychiatrist recorded an opening and closing message about stigma and provided a phone number that listeners could call for more information. The center of the message included one of three first-person accounts from people living with schizophrenia. The radio segments were aired on local stations for two weeks during the morning and afternoon commuting times. Staff reported that the radio spots generated dozens of phone calls, and many colleagues reported that they had heard the messages (Sartorius and Schulze, 2005).

More formal quantitative evaluation of the campaign was also done. Pre-test ($n = 849$) and post-test ($n = 804$) public opinion surveys were conducted to assess changes in knowledge and social distance (Stuart and Arboleda-Flórez, 2001). When asked if they had heard or seen any advertising or promotions about schizophrenia, approximately one in three could recall a radio advertisement in the post-survey compared to virtually none in the pre-survey. This indicated that the radio intervention had successfully reached a significant number of listeners. To everyone's great disappointment, however, there were no differences in knowledge or social distance scores from pre- to post-test (Sartorius and Schulze, 2005).

Figure 10.1 shows the knowledge scores for the individuals who indicated they had heard something on the radio pertaining to schizophrenia. The box represents the interquartile range (25th to 75th percentile); the midpoint reflects the median score, and the whiskers reflect the outermost scores. The median knowledge score shifted during the post-test to reflect a small improvement in knowledge. However, this did not reach statistical significance, indicating that it could have occurred by chance. Creating, producing, airing, and evaluating the radio campaign were also the most expensive of all of the activities undertaken by the local action committee, accounting for the lion's share of the meager and hard-won budget.

A key difficulty with this campaign was that it was impossible to control or contextualize competing messages that people received from other sources. For example, during the time of this campaign, negative news stories in the local newspaper increased by 25% and their word count increased by 100%. The greatest increase in negative news concerned stories about schizophrenia, the target of the radio campaign. Stigmatizing stories about schizophrenia increased by 46%, and their length increased over threefold (from 300 to 1000 words per story per month). Many of these stories were from elsewhere, but were highly charged and received considerable local, national, and international coverage. At the time of the campaign, the Unabomber trial was in full swing, and there had been several incidents in Canada and the United States of people with untreated schizophrenia committing acts of violence. One highly

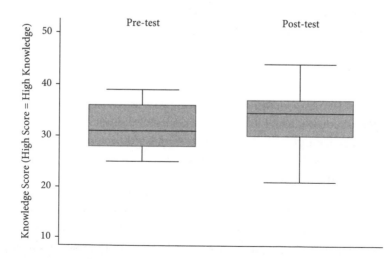

Figure 10.1 Pre-test and post-test knowledge scores following a radio campaign for those who remembered hearing a radio advertisement about schizophrenia.

visible story involved a Toronto man who pushed a commuter from a subway platform. In another, a man had sneaked into the residence of the prime minister. The front-page newspaper picture showed the prime minister with his hands around the man's neck. Our inability to control or manage the "CNN effect" was a major disadvantage of our local efforts and one key reason for the lack of population-level change (Stuart, 2003a).

A second difficulty pertained to the evaluation. The simple pre- and post-test evaluation required two representative population surveys, which were expensive and had to be contracted out to a survey firm. A comparison group would have strengthened the design, but because the entire population was targeted, no comparison group was possible. Thus, if changes had occurred, it would have been impossible to know whether they could be attributed to the program or some other extraneous event.

CAN SOCIAL INCLUSION BE SOLD LIKE SOAP?

The idea of using commercial marketing techniques to improve social conditions dates back to the middle of the twentieth century. Public health practitioners and health behavior experts fully adopted this technology to address a host of health issues, ranging from family planning, to obesity, to tobacco control, such that social marketing now occupies a central position in most public health toolkits (Stead, Hastings, and McDermott, 2007). It is also the dream of most anti-stigma groups to launch an all-out media barrage with television commercials produced by award-winning directors, speaking engagements with talk show celebrities, and news segments by acclaimed journalists (Sartorius and Schulze, 2005). This raises an important question: Can social inclusion be sold like soap or breakfast cereal?

Several benchmark criteria have been widely accepted in the field to define social marketing interventions. A summary of these and the problems that arise when using social marketing interventions to reduce prejudice and discrimination are summarized in Table 10-1.

Commercial marketing exists to change behaviors by offering an exchange. The consumer benefits by obtaining a needed or desired product in exchange for money, thereby meeting the twin goals of customer satisfaction and profit. What makes the exchange work is that each party wants something that the other has. Social marketing lacks this quid pro quo. Social marketing campaigns provide information with the aim of changing behaviors, but they are not done in exchange for behavioral change; consequently, important incentives are often lacking. Social marketers tend to view success, not in terms of behavioral change, but in terms of changed attitudes or intentions to change. In the context of commercial

Table 10-1. BENCHMARK CRITERIA FOR COMMERCIAL MARKETING AND PROBLEMS
WITH APPLICATIONS TO STIGMA REDUCTION INTERVENTIONS

Benchmark	Explanation	Problems for Anti-stigma Work
Behavior change	The goal is behavior change and there are specific, measurable objectives	Interventions focus on intermediate variables (attitudes), not on behavioral change, and have no measurable outcomes
Exchange	There are clear benefits offered in exchange for behavior change	There are no clear personal benefits in exchange for behavior change
Consumer research	Intervention is based on a clear understanding of audience values, needs, and experiences	Understanding of audience characteristics is often incomplete or unavailable
Segmentation and targeting	Audiences are segmented and target groups carefully selected	Programs are population-based and aim for universal coverage
Marketing mix	The intervention is tailored to the target groups selected	Messages are not tailored to target groups selected
Competition	Analyze sources of competing messages and set strategies to remove or minimize these	There are powerful, negative competing media messages and social structures that create and maintain stigma and social exclusion

See Stead, Hastings, and McDermott (2007) for a more detailed description of the
benchmarks and their explanation.

marketing, this would be akin to increasing the number of people who would
consider becoming customers in the future (Peattie and Peattie, 2003).

Instead of selling goods or services, social marketers must sell propositions
that may, or in the case of broader social goods, may not, have a direct or tangible benefit to their audience. Within this context, stigma reduction and social
inclusion are hard commodities to sell, particularly when there are powerful
social forces that can easily overwhelm positive marketing messages, and when
there is no clear personal benefit to the individual. Indeed, in light of the enduring stereotype of dangerousness and the nightly barrage of media and news
messages reinforcing the idea that people with a mental illness are dangerous
and unpredictable, most people would consider the benefit of maintaining a
safe distance (Stuart, 2003b).

It is also arguable that anti-stigma campaigns have not shown fidelity to key marketing principles, which require a sophisticated psychographic understanding of the audience in order to tailor and target messages. The message and the techniques of a campaign often dominate the agenda, rather than the nature, needs, or likely responses of target audiences. Campaigns are launched without any prior research and even despite prior research. Mental health literacy campaigns that are directed to audiences that are already highly literate are one such example. Rather than focusing on what people should know or think, campaigners would do well to develop a better understanding of what specific behaviors need to change and what incentives need to be in place to make these changes possible. This can only be determined by asking people who bear the burden of stigma—an area that is significantly under-researched.

Over-reliance on familiar tools and inadequate attention to the principles and challenges of social marketing as applied to stigma reduction have led to a situation where it is the message and the needs of those communicating the message that have dominated the agenda; not the nature, needs, or responses of target audiences (Peattie and Peattie, 2003). The focus on individual-level change has also diverted attention from addressing the important structural components of stigma. Andreasen (2002) has argued for an increased role for social marketing aimed at structural forces, such as policy makers, media, lawmakers, or educators, and Morris and Clarkson (2009) have suggested that a social marketing framework could be used to improve the implementation of clinical practice guidelines by physicians.

Because social marketing approaches work best when targeting discrete behavioral change involving a clear benefit, they may be better suited to achieving literacy-based goals, such as improving help-seeking behaviors. Corrigan and colleagues (Corrigan, Roe, and Tsang, 2011) have suggested that marketing campaigns may have their greatest influence on label-avoidance behaviors when they illustrate and legitimize the suffering attached to mental illnesses and direct people to local mental health services or web links where they can obtain additional information. However, the effectiveness of this application will have to wait for future testing.

Even if social marketing campaigns were implemented with greater fidelity to marketing principles, it is unlikely that they would be potent enough to change the power structures that serve to entrench social inequities experienced by people with a mental illness. Indeed, in the absence of structural changes, it is unlikely that any educational effort alone could remove structural barriers that reduce life chances for people with a mental illness. In many parts of Europe, for example, people with a mental illness are experiencing a trend toward re-institutionalization following the closure of long-stay mental hospitals in the 1980s. Characteristics of this trend include increasing

mechanisms for risk-containment through forensic or civil commitment procedures. Investments in confinement are taking the place of investments in
supports for civic participation (Sayce and Curran, 2005). Also, because discrimination is a pervasive and persistent phenomenon, attempts to change it
in one area will almost certainly mean that it will emerge in another under a
different guise. Consequently, initiatives need to be multifaceted and multi-
level (Link and Phelan, 2001).

Finally, in our increasingly multicultural societies, it can be impossible to
craft media images and messages that are acceptable to all cultural groups.
What may be viewed as a positive message for one group may be offensive for
another. When developing media messages for an information campaign on
employment, a Berlin-based firm found it challenging to come up with images
that worked across race, gender, disability, age, sexual, and religious groups.
They finally settled on an image of robots in the office to highlight the importance of diversity; however, it is unlikely that this generic and politically correct
offering would improve the hiring practices of employers or reduce workplace
stigma directed toward workers with a mental illness (Sayce and Curran, 2005).
Perhaps, then, we need to be more thoughtful and selective in our use of social
marketing and consider that it might not be the best tool to fight prejudice or
discrimination.

In summary, there are many limitations to universal anti-stigma campaigns,
which mainly rely on mass media to get messages across to the lay public.
Population-based campaigns tend to be expensive, therefore of limited duration. As well as being expensive to implement, they are expensive to evaluate.
Even if they lead to changes in knowledge or attitudes, it is unlikely that they are
potent enough to create social structures that are more inclusive of people with
a mental illness, or to change behavior.

11

Paradigm 10: Mental Illnesses Are Like Any Other Illnesses

any anti-stigma programs are built on the premise that mental ill-nesses are like any other illnesses, and once the public realizes the similarities between mental illnesses and other physical conditions, they will adopt a more benevolent view. However, mental illnesses are not like other illnesses. Historical and political realities have made them different. Also, the way in which they express themselves is different in that, above all, they affect social relations and functioning. To overlook these fundamental facts is to deeply misunderstand the nature and effects of stigma attached to mental illnesses.

FORCED CONFINEMENT AND TREATMENT

Mental illnesses are not like other illnesses, because they regularly cause people to lose their rights and freedoms in ways that are unimaginable in other health conditions. Mental illnesses may also be expressed in behaviors that are objectionable to others. The psychiatric profession is one of only three groups in modern societies that have the authority to remove an individual's freedom; the other two being judges, following police apprehension in the case of a crime; and medical officers of health, following quarantine procedures in the case of an outbreak. Szasz (2007) defined psychiatry as the *theory and practice of coercion* and suggested that it is the legally authorized paternalism that distinguishes psychiatry from all other branches of medicine.

Historically, the care of the mentally ill has been deplorable. During the great confinement in the early part of the 1800s, hospital officials in Europe had the authority to round up and imprison people who were mentally ill (termed then *madmen* and *idiots*), along with beggars, vagabonds, criminals, the unemployed, and other undesirables. The characterization of the mentally ill as wild beasts justified their forcible confinement and social banishment. In some parts of Europe, people with a mental illness were cast adrift in the now legendary *ships of fools*, never to be allowed safe port (Arboleda-Flórez, 2008). It is sobering to realize that most countries still rely on custodial institutions for the confinement and treatment of the mentally ill. The government policy of many countries is to put people with mental illnesses in large institutions that are situated in remote parts of the country where they will have little or no contact with the outside world, save through the staff. A 2003 report of conditions in the European Union indicates that in both Central and Eastern Europe, there are numerous large residential institutions with unacceptable conditions and human rights violations (European Research Initiative on Community-Based Residential Alternatives for Disabled People, 2003). Individuals are placed in these institutions involuntarily without due-process safeguards or the right to have their cases reviewed. The institutions are unhygienic and poorly maintained. The residents live in large overcrowded dormitories with insufficient food, with no facilities to keep personal possessions, and no rehabilitative or therapeutic activities. It was conservatively estimated that some 2,354 institutions are in operation across 29 countries with almost 200,000 residents. In some countries, such as Austria, 70% of residents have been institutionalized for more than a decade. In most cases, a third to one-half of the residents are long-stay. In some institutions in Romania, Hungary, and France, the typical length of stay is for life.

In 2003, Krosnar reported that mentally ill patients in four Central European countries (preparing to join the European Union) were being kept in padlocked, caged beds (Figure 11.1). In some cases, the patients had been locked in the beds for months or years, and sometimes not even let out to use the toilet. Several, including one fourteen-year-old girl, had died. Despite widespread condemnation of the practice by the European Parliament, the United Nations, and patients' rights organizations, some doctors indicated that the use of cage beds was justified under certain circumstances and in light of the lack of resources (including staff) available to provide therapeutic alternatives (Krosnar, 2003).

In modern psychiatric systems, psychiatrists continue to apply police power in criminal proceedings and through civil commitment legislation that allows for involuntary hospitalization and, increasingly, community-based commitments. As the locus of care has switched from the hospital to the community, so have commitment laws. "Community treatment orders" have emerged as one of the most controversial issues in modern mental health policy. Critics argue that mandated treatment is counterproductive and likely to result in adverse reactions such as failing to engage in treatment and avoiding future treatment for fear of coercion. Proponents argue that mandated treatment is effective and may help restore an individual's ability to make rational, autonomous decisions. Empirical results show that a third or more of patients fear

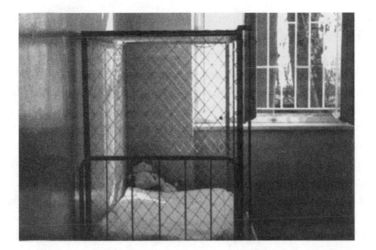

Figure 11.1 Cage beds used to confine patients in Central Europe (*Source*: Mental Disability Advocacy Center. Cage Beds: inhuman and degrading treatment or punishment in four EU accession countries. Budapest: Mental Disability Advocacy Center; 2003. With permission from Mental Disability Advocacy Center.).

coerced treatment and that this is a barrier to help-seeking (Swartz, Swanson, and Hannon, 2003).

Coercion is not restricted to involuntary patients. In studying a consecutive series of voluntary and involuntary patients in two Swedish counties, Eriksson and Westrin (1995) found that one-third of the voluntary patients and two-thirds of the involuntary patients reported the occurrence of coercive measures during their admission. Being locked in was the most frequent example of restraint among both groups. Voluntary patients also noted threats of legal commitment. Over half of the committed patients and 38% of the voluntary patients reported that they had felt violated as a human being. These results demonstrate an important gray area between voluntariness and coercion in modern psychiatric care.

ANTI-PSYCHIATRY SENTIMENTS

Dain (1989) suggests that religious, political, scientific, and intellectual forces have converged to put psychiatry on the defensive in a way that is unlike any other professional group. It would be highly unlikely to see protests and placard-waving antagonists picketing outside of a medical conference, yet this has become routine for psychiatric conferences. Busloads of protesters often attend large psychiatric association conferences with banners that contain slogans such as "*Psychiatry Kills.*" In some countries, protesters are confined to an area where they cannot disturb conference attendees. In others, they line the main avenue to the congress center—as unruly mobs—requiring conference participants walk the gauntlet to enter the main doors, during which time they are shouted at, cursed, spat at, jostled, and have leaflets thrust into their faces. The protesters bring drums and loudspeakers and create as much noise as possible in the hope of disrupting the meetings. In some conferences, enterprising anti-psychiatry enthusiasts set up parallel exhibitions in nearby locations so that conference-goers can (for a small fee) be educated about past and current atrocities committed by modern psychiatry and psychiatrists. It is difficult to imagine a similar display at a conference devoted to the care and management of cancer or diabetes.

Psychiatry must be one of the most criticized and misunderstood medical professions. Indeed, even the term *survivor* is used differently—not as a cancer survivor would—but in the same menacing way that one would refer to a *rape survivor* or a *Holocaust survivor*, as someone who has survived a traumatic event at the hands of abusers—in this case, coercive psychiatric treatment (Torrey, 2010).

The World Psychiatric Association's Task Force on the Destigmatization of Psychiatry and Psychiatrists reports that public opinion about psychiatry and psychiatric treatments has been largely negative, based on misconceptions about psychotropic medications such as: they are addictive, a form of sedation without cure, an invasion of identity, mere drugging of patients, or ineffective in preventing relapse. Negative opinions about electroconvulsive therapy and psychiatric hospitals are also widespread. The public image of psychiatrists shows a lack of knowledge about the nature and extent of their medical training (e.g., not believing they are "real" medical doctors) and misperceptions about their role as "agents of repression" whose purpose is to guarantee conformity, "see into people's minds," or create "loopholes for criminals." Psychiatrists have been viewed as "dangerous and manipulative abusers who exploit their patients and abuse their power, even to the extent of trying to obtain sexual favours" (Sartorius et al., 2010, p. 134).

Though many branches of medicine have been criticized, their very existence has not been disputed through attacks from within their own ranks. Crossley (1998) makes the point that a key feature of the anti-psychiatry movement that distinguished it from other critical currents at the time was that it was a *revolt from above*. It was led by a small group of eminent psychiatrists who were writing during the 1960s and 1970s, such as Cooper and Laing in England, Szasz in the United States, and Bassaglia in Italy. Though the term *anti-psychiatry* was originally coined by Cooper to designate a critical perspective that was taken from within psychiatry, it was subsequently used more widely to refer to broader criticisms of organized psychiatry that emerged during the 1960s and 1970s, including the consumer-survivor movement and the Church of Scientology.

Though specific theories diverge considerably, a central organizing theme of the critics has been the sharp rejection of the medical model, shared views that organized psychiatry is an agent of social control and that psychiatric illness is product of the struggle between a repressive society and a nonconforming individual. From this perspective, the genesis of mental illness is considered to be entirely social, with no underlying biological basis. Psychiatry is seen as an entirely a political weapon focused on restraining civil liberties. Its job is to medicalize defiance and persecute nonconformists. Widespread use of involuntary hospitalization and forced treatment in the United States, and the historical use of psychiatry as a measure to deal with political dissidents in the Soviet Union, provided stark examples (Nasser, 1995).

Consumer-survivor groups, which emerged as early as the turn of the last century, have played an important role in drawing attention to the human rights issues raised by involuntary and coercive treatment. Former patients have provided some of the earliest and most radical critiques of psychiatric authority. Indeed, the mental health field has produced some of the most radical and angry patient movements. During the 1970s, many consumer groups drew from the intellectual traditions of the anti-psychiatry movement, particularly the work of Laing and Szasz, which questioned the very existence of mental illnesses. Their aim was not so much to influence mental health reforms, but to develop viable alternatives to the mental health system that embraced core principals such as overturning medical authority, promoting self-determination, and resisting stereotypes (Tomes, 2006).

Ex-patient groups expressed considerable hurt and anger. They denied that the treatments they had been provided within the mental health system were effective or appropriate, and they forcefully proclaimed that they were the best qualified to judge whether and how they should be treated. They established their own self-help programs as alternatives to hospitals and community-based programs. There was also resentment against a profession that had the power to brand them as "mentally disabled," and the human rights issues surrounding the practice of involuntary commitment remained a deep concern (Dain, 1989).

The Church of Scientology epitomizes the anti-psychiatry movement and has used its financial and other resources to wage media campaigns against psychiatry and the pharmaceutical industry. Public demonstrations and critiques by celebrities such as Tom Cruise have questioned organized psychiatry's views of mental illnesses and treatment approaches (Sharfstein and Dickerson, 2006). Scientologists' extremist views oppose psychiatric treatments, which they consider brutal, inhumane, and inefficacious. Scientology doctrine also bans reaching out for help from organized psychiatry. Instead, it offers its own brand of self-improvement and psychotherapy in an effort to draw people with mental illnesses into the church (*Psychiatric Times*, 1991). As a result of anti-psychiatry sentiments, the voices of service users are increasingly incorporated into mental health services planning and research, and system outcomes are more often defined in terms that emphasize social inclusion, rather than amelioration of symptoms.

VIOLENCE AND UNPREDICTABILITY

The public perception of people with a mental illness as violent and unpredictable dramatically sets them apart from people with other health conditions. No other medical condition is so intertwined with issues of violence and dangerousness in the public's eyes. People with a mental illness are not generally viewed as benign or in need of social support, but are more often considered a public risk. The general public most fear violence that is random and unpredictable—the kind of violence that is regularly portrayed by media as the kind perpetrated by the mentally ill. Public perceptions of violence and risk of violence are central to their support for coercive treatments, legislative solutions, and justifications for social inequities and injustices. High rates of victimization among people with a mental illness go unnoticed (Stuart, 2003b).

Over time, there has been a progressive convergence of mental illness and violence in clinical practice. While researchers and clinicians initially disavowed any relationship, there has been a growing willingness by professionals to accept the violence stereotype and to see their professional role as one of predicting and managing violent behaviors. Most mental health professionals can report personal experiences of physical violence at the hands of a patient. The widespread adoption of the dangerousness standard as the basis for civil commitment and the reduction in hospital beds noted in many developed countries means that only those who are at highest risk of violence will ever be admitted as an inpatient.

A random sample of almost 1,500 Americans responding to the General Social Survey were asked to consider five vignettes describing a person with: alcohol dependence, major depression, schizophrenia, drug dependence, and emotional troubles. Figure 11.2 shows the proportion of respondents who indicated that the person in the vignette was "very likely" or "somewhat likely" to do something violent to others. It also shows the proportion who agreed to involuntary commitment if the individual was a danger to others. As these results illustrate, the public discriminate between different types of mental health problems by their likelihood of dangerousness and greatly exaggerate

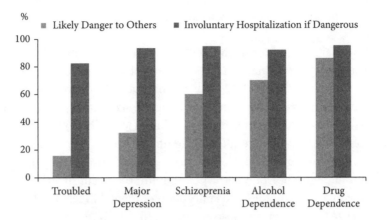

Figure 11.2 Public perceptions of dangerousness, and support for involuntary hospitalization. (*Source*: Pescosolido, B., Monahan, J., Link, B., Stueve, A., and Kikuzawa, S. (1999). The Public's View of the Competence, Dangerousness, and Need for Legal Coercion of Persons with Mental Health Problems. *American Journal of Public Health*, *89*, 1339–1345.).

the risk. Based on inaccurate and exaggerated perceptions of threat, members of the public are entirely supportive of coerced treatment of people with mental illnesses through involuntary hospitalization when they think dangerousness is at issue. Though not shown in this figure, the same was true if the respondent was deemed to be a danger to self.

AN ILLNESS LIKE ANY OTHER?

With growing understanding of the genetic and neurobiological components of mental illnesses, the theoretical basis for the anti-psychiatry movement (emphasizing the exclusively social genesis of mental illnesses) is being eroded. Many advocates now believe that stigma could be reduced if we could educate people that mental illnesses are brain disorders—real biological diseases, like any other. In fact, stigma reduction efforts using information about the biological bases for mental illnesses have become a mainstay of many policy recommendations and international efforts, and there have been efforts since the 1990s to educate the public about the biological causes of mental illnesses.

The problem with saying that mental illnesses are like any other is that, based on what they see on the nightly news, the public is deeply aware that mental illnesses are not like any other. Moreover, the persistence with which this message has been conveyed has significantly eroded the credibility of organized psychiatry and mental health advocacy. The public has lost confidence in the messengers.

The National Alliance for the Mentally Ill in the United States has been particularly active in disseminating results of research on biological causes of serious mental illness (Phelan, 2005). Also, a number of literacy programs have been developed to assist people in identifying the signs and symptoms of mental illnesses so as to foster greater help seeking (Jorm, 2000). However, while these intensive efforts have resulted in significant and widespread increases in public understanding of biological theories and improved public support for treatment, there has been no corresponding improvement in social tolerance. In fact, holding a neurobiological conception of mental illness has been shown to be unrelated to stigma, and worse, it has been shown to increase the odds of a stigmatizing reaction (Pescosolido, Martin, Long, Medina, and Link, 2010). A competing explanation that seems to have received insufficient attention is that an illness model may lead to the belief that people will have no control over their behavior, and that since the illness has affected the brain structure, they will not recover, thereby increasing widespread fears centering on dangerousness and unpredictability.

In our experiences, mental illnesses as "brain diseases" are even less well received in Europe than in the United States. For example, Dietrich and colleagues examined the relationship between biological causal beliefs and social distance from people with schizophrenia and depression, and found that explanations that centered on brain disease and heredity were consistently associated with higher levels of social distance in Germany, Russia, and Mongolia. They suggest that their findings provide an impetus to reconsider the assumption underlying many anti-stigma interventions: that promulgating biological concepts among the public will reduce social distance (Dietrich, Beck, Bujantugs, Kenzine, Matschinger, and Angermeyer, 2004).

Haslam, Sayce, and Davies (2006) reviewed the literature published between 1970 and 2004 and identified 21 studies that examined the relationship between lay etiological theories of mental illnesses and negative attitudes. They found a steady stream of research linking biological explanations to negative and stigmatizing attitudes. Of the 19 associations between biological explanations and stigmatizing attitudes tested in these publications, all but one were negative. Conversely, of the 12 associations between psychological explanations and mental illnesses, all but one were positive. Biological explanations were also more likely to be associated with stereotypes of dangerousness and unpredictability. Mental health professionals who subscribed to the biological perspective were less likely to involve patients in service planning. These results were consistent across countries: the United States, Hong Kong, New Zealand, Australia, East Germany, West Germany, Russia, and Mongolia. Four studies demonstrated that challenging biological theories reduced social distance and stereotyping among adolescents and young adults. This is overwhelming evidence that the "illness like any other" or the "disease view" engenders negative and stigmatizing attitudes and should not be used as the basis for anti-stigma efforts.

The increasing prominence of genetic explanations for health conditions may further exacerbate this situation by reinforcing the notion that someone with a mental illness is fundamentally (genetically) different from others, that the problem is serious and persistent, and that it is likely to occur within the family. Genetic explanations for mental illnesses have been demonstrated to be associated with increased social distance, particularly with regard to more intimate relationships (Phelan, 2005), and in the early days of the asylum, the assumed genetic taint went hand in hand with negative views of prognosis and social segregation (Shortt, 1986). The idea that mental illnesses are genetically determined led to passivity and pessimism about treatment, particularly at the turn of the century. Freud's influence made it possible to have hope. In Freud's view, the causes of mental illnesses were not external and immutable, thus leading to the idea that something could be done to resolve them.

In conclusion, we would argue that mental illnesses are not like any other illnesses. The unique socio-political history that has centered on coercive treatment has culminated in strong anti-psychiatry currents that do not afflict other medical conditions. Public perceptions that exaggerate the risk of violence, the need for segregation, and the use of involuntary confinement also set mental illnesses apart. Finally, although biological explanations for mental illnesses have gained prominence, their use in anti-stigma programs has been associated with increased social intolerance. Anti-stigma programs that promote the "illness like any other" message may do more harm than good.

12

Paradigm 11: Stigma Can't Be Beaten

I t is easy to believe that stigma is so deeply engrained in our social fabric that no program could prevent or reduce it. It may be that stigma has been difficult to budge because we have been using the wrong approaches. This chapter will challenge the belief that "stigma can't be beaten", using examples from the literature as well as our own experiences to highlight promising practices.

THE IMPORTANCE OF FIGHTING BACK

In 2001, at the 54th World Health Assembly, the World Health Organization called on health ministers to redress mental health–related disparities (WHO, 2001). This was preceded by a number of resolutions of the World Health Assembly and other governing bodies of WHO (Sartorius, 2002c) and followed by a global advocacy program that was initiated for World Health Day in 2003 (WHO, 2001) and a global action program to raise awareness of the importance of mental health (WHO, 2003). International support for anti-stigma efforts was also evident when, in 2004, the Council of European Ministers pledged support for anti-stigma activities in a special ministerial meeting convened by the Ministry of Health of Greece within the framework of the Greek presidency of the European Union (Stefanis and Economou, 2005).

Prestigious international organizations such as the World Health Organization, the World Psychiatric Association, and the World Association of Social Psychiatry have identified stigma as the single most important challenge to mental health reform. The World Psychiatric Association's *Open the Doors* program, which began work in 1996, was the first international attempt to fight stigma and discrimination. Members of the program subsequently organized a series of international *Together Against Stigma* congresses, which have been held in Leipzig, Germany (in 2001); Kingston, Canada (in 2003); Istanbul, Turkey (in 2006); and London (in 2009). In addition, in 2005, the World Psychiatric

Association's General Assembly approved the development of a scientific section on stigma and mental disorders, which has drawn together scientists and practitioners from around the world with the common goal of developing best practices to eliminate the stigma associated with mental illnesses. Finally, in 2009, the president of the World Psychiatric Association established a task force and entrusted it with the development of a guidance paper on how to combat the stigmatization of psychiatry and psychiatrists (Sartorius et al., 2010).

The rise in public health models focusing on the burden of mental illnesses and their social determinants, and the corresponding ascendancy of anti-stigma programs, marks an important conceptual shift. Previously, mental illnesses were largely excluded from public health programs. While this situation has improved, mental illnesses are not yet seen in the same way, or given the same importance, as other chronic or disabling conditions. This is exemplified by the fact that in September of 2011, the United Nations devoted a special session to the problems of non-communicable diseases, because of their importance for national development, but excluded mental illnesses from their agenda.

The last two decades have marked the coming of age for anti-stigma programming worldwide and international support for anti-stigma efforts is increasing. Throughout this book we have argued that smaller, focused efforts that are more sustainable are preferable to large, universally targeted campaigns. The following are examples of targeted approaches to anti-stigma activities that have shown promise.

OVERCOMING NIMBYISM—THE "NOT IN MY BACK YARD" SYNDROME

In Chapter 2 we identified the NIMBY syndrome as a significant barrier to placing mental health supports and services within local communities. Overcoming NIMBYism is an important means of improving housing options and other community supports required by people with a mental illness to foster social participation and community life. Research has shown that carefully targeted neighborhood programs using elements of social contact can make an important difference.

In 1993, staffed group houses were opened in two areas in West Lambeth as part of the closure of Tooting Bec Hospital—a large Victorian-era asylum in South London. The neighbors in one area received a targeted educational program, including a didactic component (an information package containing a video and fact sheets), a social component (social events and social overtures from staff), and a mixed component (a formal reception with formal discussion sessions). One year following the educational program, neighbors in the area that received this program were significantly more likely to make contact with staff; know the names of staff and count them among their friends; know the names of the residents of the group houses; and have social interaction with them, including visiting them, counting them as friends, and inviting them into their homes. Percentage differences were large. For example, 28% of neighbors in the experimental area reported social contact with the group home residents, compared to only 8% in the control area. No residents in the control area counted the group home residents as friends, compared to 13% in the experimental area. There were no significant differences in knowledge, suggesting that it was the social contact with staff and patients, not the educational materials themselves, that led to less-fearful attitudes (Wolf, Pathare, Craig, and Leff, 1999).

In this case, it was the attitudes of the staff, rather than those of the community residents, that threatened the success of the program, illustrating the importance of overcoming stigma in mental health professionals. Some of the staff objected to the program because they were concerned that it would draw attention to the group home residents. If the residents were not known by their neighbors to be mentally ill, and were perceived to be the same as anyone else, there should be no reason to deliberately encourage their integration into the community. Many staff members considered that the neighbors would not be interested and did not feel that the program would have any beneficial effects. It was often difficult for staff to find time to put into this project, as it was viewed as outside of their main therapeutic mandate. Finally, it also proved to be difficult to obtain ethics approval to conduct the research, because of a fear of provoking a backlash against the facilities and because of concerns about confidentiality. These issues delayed the delivery of the educational program until after the houses were opened. Neighbors would have liked more information earlier, and some considered that there was too much secrecy surrounding the opening of the houses.

This example supports the effectiveness of personal contact—in this case achieved through social events—and the importance of ensuring that professional stereotypes do not get in the way of service delivery. Mental health clinicians have come late to the issue of stigma reduction, and many view it as something outside of their appropriate range of activities. The study also highlights the importance of early intervention with neighborhoods targeted for community based programs so as to disarm the vocal minority that may otherwise sway neighborhood sentiments.

CHANGING THE WAY EMERGENCY DEPARTMENTS DO BUSINESS

Emergency rooms in hospitals (emergency departments) are among the environments in which the stigma of mental illnesses is generated with particularly bad effects. Changing the way in which emergency departments do business is, therefore, an important anti-stigma goal. In 1998, a team working under the auspices of the Canadian Pilot Project of the World Psychiatric Association's *Open the Doors* global anti-stigma program interviewed local patients and family members concerning issues that were pertinent to the emergency care of people with a mental illness: such as privacy, security, policies on patient rights, use of restraints, wait times, staff training, and satisfaction with services (Sartorius and Schulze, 2005). At the time, local health systems were undergoing significant restructuring and reform, including some capital construction, so there was an important window of opportunity in which to act. Results were presented and discussed with the administrators of each local hospital with an eye to improving emergency practices.

Two of the four hospitals were considered to have adequate space to provide private and secure services for people presenting with a mental health crisis. Two of the hospitals did not. Three of the hospitals had policies governing patients' rights, but the way in which this information was provided to patients and their families differed. Similarly, not all of the hospitals had clear policies on the use of restraints. Three of the four emergency departments had access to specialty psychiatric staff, but these individuals were not available at all times. Similarly, training for emergency staff in the management of mental health crisis varied. None of the hospitals had wait-time data to assess whether psychiatric patients were waiting longer (or inordinately longer) than other patients, and no hospital had data describing the satisfaction of psychiatric patients and their families with the emergency care received—therefore, there were clear gaps in the quality assessment process.

At the close of the project, none of the hospitals had a comprehensive plan to address the issues raised. The evaluation team recognized that broader standards would be required to facilitate this process, so they contacted the national hospital accrediting body. The items from the local survey were recast and included in the hospital accreditation survey that subsequently would be used to evaluate all hospitals in Canada, illustrating the importance of considering structural changes to important policies and practices as an anti-stigma tool. The accreditation criteria used are shown in Figure 12.1.

CONNECTING WITH TEACHERS AND STUDENTS

Considerable research has now supported the use of contact-based education involving people with a mental illness telling their personal stories. School-based programs using contact-based education have been a central and effective

1. The examination and interview process and space are adequate for the safety, security and privacy of patients and staff.
2. There are enough private interview rooms available to ensure privacy during interviews in most situations.
3. Interview rooms are secure.
4. Security staff are available on a timely, as need, basis.
5. There is a policy in place governing the use of restraints.

Figure 12.1 Special accreditation guidelines for patients with a mental illness.

feature of many anti-stigma activities worldwide (Sartorius and Schulze, 2005). Typically, these programs are organized and delivered by local advocacy groups and are conducted on a shoestring budget with little or no financial support from mental health agencies. Speakers usually undergo some training in public speaking, but this may vary. Because trained speakers may not be available in all communities, and the skill set of local speakers may vary, the question of whether a video-based intervention could work as well has been raised. Videos provide standardized interventions and are more easily disseminated.

Chan and colleagues (2009) compared the effects of three forms of education targeting high school students' perceptions of people with schizophrenia in Hong Kong. The first condition was a traditional demythologizing lecture (traditional education). In the second condition, the lecture was followed by a contact video; and in the third condition, the contact video was provided first, followed by the lecture. All classes were led by a clinical psychologist trainee. The video featured four real people (two males and two females) who had been diagnosed with schizophrenia in early adulthood. They all had made a good recovery; living independently with jobs and a good quality of life. They shared their experiences with symptoms and talked about stigma and how they overcame it to regain a fulfilling life. Ten classes of Grade 9 students participated in the project. Classes in each school were randomly assigned to one of the conditions. Measures were collected before, just after, and one month following the classes. Participants in the group that received the educational session followed by the video demonstrated improved attitudes and reduced social distance toward someone with schizophrenia—an effect that was still evident at the one-month follow-up, though smaller. Students in the other two groups did not show any improvements. Based on these findings, researchers were able to develop a kit of educational materials that was provided to over 600 secondary schools throughout Hong Kong.

A similar video-plus-contact educational program was developed by the Schizophrenia Society of Canada. It involved lesson plans and teaching materials for two full classes to be taught by the regular classroom teacher. In the first lesson, students learned about schizophrenia and were given an opportunity to share their knowledge. This was followed by a 20-minute video introducing the signs and symptoms of schizophrenia, using a dramatization of a student who was worried about a friend's behavior, and the real-life experiences of five individuals who had schizophrenia. Students then participated in an active discussion about their response to the video, reviewed basic facts, and clarified any misunderstandings. They learned about the major myths, the early warning signs, the role of stigma as a barrier to help-seeking and recovery, and what to do if a friend showed signs of schizophrenia. In the second lesson, students role-played to reinforce the messages of the first lesson. Lessons were accompanied by questionnaires, answer sheets, discussion questions, presentation templates, and ideas for further active learning.

This program was evaluated in eight high schools across Canada ($n = 571$) (Stuart, 2006c). Knowledge and attitude scores were calculated using standard questionnaires, and the proportion of students achieving 80% or more correct answers formed the basis for the impact assessment. At baseline, 48% of the students included in the evaluation had achieved 80% or higher on the knowledge questions. This improved to 79% on the post test, reflecting a large and statistically significant change. Similarly, 42% of the students exceeded the threshold on the social tolerance items at baseline, rising to 52% at follow-up, reflecting a smaller, but still statistically significant difference. In responses to open-ended questions, 25% of the students reported the main take-home message they learned was that schizophrenia was treatable. Thirteen percent reported that they had learned that they held false stereotypes concerning violence and dangerousness.

This program is important because it provided supports for teachers to engage students. It combined indirect video contact with active learning and role-playing over two lessons. The magnitude of the changes documented was comparable to those of high school programs that used direct contact with someone who had schizophrenia. The strengths of a video presentation combined with opportunities for active learning, compared to direct personal contact, include greater cost-effectiveness, feasibility, and standardization.

As a cautionary note, it is important to ensure that video content does not portray negative or stereotypical images of people with a mental illness. Rather, the images must be of someone who has recovered from an illness and who is successfully managing their day-to-day lives. It is also desirable if the people portrayed on the video are similar to the target audience in age and appearance. Otherwise, negative stereotypes may be vividly consolidated and stigma increased. As part of an anti-stigma program in Toronto, for example, high school students were shown a video that depicted the challenges faced by homeless individuals who were mentally ill (Tolomiczenko, Goering, and Durbin, 2001). The video featured caseworkers, clients, and psychiatrists who described a case management program for mentally ill homeless persons designed to improve their residential stability, reduce psychiatric symptoms, and improve social functioning. On the video, clients spoke about their illness, homelessness, and recovery. Staff talked about the program and its goals. It portrayed life on the street and the paths taken toward housing and mental stability. Students who viewed the video showed more negative attitudes on all of the scales and reported stronger feelings of danger associated with homeless persons. They also endorsed more restrictions. Those who viewed the video and had time for discussion had lower stigma scores on two of the four scales, and were less likely to view homeless people through a lens of dangerousness. The chronicling of the housing struggles of these individuals, without an adequate opportunity for discussion, intensified negative feelings and entrenched stigma.

ENGAGING THE POLICE

Police officers are important first responders to many mental health crises, and they have discretionary judgment that allows them to take someone in crisis to hospital or to a jail. In the post-deinstitutionalization era, police have increasing contact with people who have a mental illness and are living in the community. Unfortunately, police have little formal training in mental health, leaving them at risk of overreacting in metal health emergencies. All too often we hear of fatal shootings or taser incidents involving someone with a mental illness. This has led a number of anti-stigma programs to target police.

An organized course targeting police officers was mounted in Boulder, Colorado, as part of the World Psychiatric Association's *Open the Doors* program (Leff and Warner, 2006). Mental health professionals, consumers, and police officers collaborated in developing an eight-hour training program provided to all officers in the county's largest city. Training was delivered on six occasions, each time to a portion of the force. The content was delivered by psychiatrists, family members, and people with a mental illness. Pre- and post-testing showed a 48% improvement in basic knowledge (myths and facts about schizophrenia) and a 13% improvement in knowledge of the causes of schizophrenia. Smaller improvements (11%) were noted with respect to officers' beliefs about the usual behavior of people with schizophrenia. Although knowledge improved, after training, 71% of the officers still believed that people with schizophrenia were always irrational, more likely than the average person to be violent, and usually unable to make life decisions. Police encounters with people with psychoses most often occur when the individual is acutely disturbed and illustrating some or all of these behaviors. This suggested that police training must include much more intensive and extensive exposure to people who have recovered from psychosis who are working and in stable relationships.

Pinfold and colleagues (Pinfold, Huxley, Thornicroft, Farmer, Toulmin, and Graham, 2003) delivered a brief contact-based educational intervention to police in Kent, in southeast England. The intervention was delivered by service users, family caregivers, and mental health professionals. Over a two-month period, police attended two workshops, each two hours in duration. Workshop sessions combined small-group work, short talks based on individuals' personal experiences, and opportunities for discussion. The first session focused on characterizing mental health problems, and the second focused on what police can do to support people with a mental health problem. Pre-test measures were collected prior to officers attending the program, and post-test measures were collected four weeks after the final training session ($n = 232$). Attitude and social distance measures were included among the measures. Paired data were available for 109 officers. Thirty-five percent of the officers admitted that they were skeptical about attending the sessions. Statistically significant improvements in attitudes were noted. In addition, there were significant improvements in the proportion of officers who recounted one of the five key workshop messages: "We all have mental health needs" (20% improvement); "People with mental health problems are far less dangerous than most people believe" (19%); "People with mental health problems can, with treatment, return to lead normal lives" (34%); "One in four people will experience a mental health problem at some point in their lives" (24%); and "Schizophrenia is not like having a split personality" (38%).

Violence was a frequent characteristic of police encounters with people who have a mental illness. At baseline, reference to violence and mental illness was a strong theme in police accounts. In the section on recording a memorable encounter, 52% recounted a violent incident, most often involving violence toward others. Overall, the session did not impact officers' beliefs about dangerousness. At baseline, 61% agreed that people with mental health problems were likely to be violent. This dropped to 54% at follow-up, but was not statistically significant in this sample. There were no differences in social distance. At baseline, 21% of the officers expressed no social distance across the four questionnaire items, and at follow-up this was 23%. At follow-up, almost 60% of the officers identified ways in which the training had made a difference to their police work (particularly in their ability to communicate with people who have a mental health problem), and 73% recommended that the educational program be delivered to other officers. Thus, despite the fact that the dangerousness stereotype proved to be more resilient than originally hoped, this intervention was able to improve self-reported behaviors and provide police with important skills and competencies that they used when dealing with mentally ill members of the public.

ENGAGING THE MEDIA

People with a mental illness and their family members are acutely aware of the negative images perpetrated by the news and entertainment media, and they blame them for perpetuating negative stereotypes and social stigma. Consequently, interventions that target negative media depictions often figure high on the list of priorities for stigma-busting activities. However, even when local media are enlisted in anti-stigma activities, the global reach of the news and entertainment media makes it difficult to stem the flow of negative imagery. Nevertheless, it is possible to enlist members of the news and entertainment media in anti-stigma activities.

In Australia, for example, producers and scriptwriters of a popular teenage soap opera with a viewing audience of 1.5 million created a storyline in which one of the main characters, Joey, experienced schizophrenia (SANE Australia, 2007). The story developed over three months. Non-stigmatizing behaviors and recovery messages were reinforced. Members of a local advocacy group (SANE Australia) and local clinicians consulted with producers and scriptwriters to ensure that the story was both realistic and positive. A helpline number was given, a chat site was created, and the actor who played Joey became involved in the publicity for the campaign. In the three months following, there was extensive national media coverage, resulting in a 100% increase in helpline and online contacts. By working with local anti-stigma programs, the show was able to illustrate how someone could recover from schizophrenia; thereby transmitting the important message that schizophrenia was treatable. They also showed how people with schizophrenia could be stigmatized and highlighted the effects of stigma on the person and family. More important, they modeled non-stigmatizing behaviors. While this example illustrates how the media may be enlisted to assist in help-seeking efforts, the effects of this television show on the knowledge, attitudes, and behaviors of the general public or the effects for people with a mental illness were never measured.

In an effort to moderate media depictions, a number of countries have implemented anti-stigma programs that target the media. For example, there are several media-monitoring projects that have been initiated by members of advocacy groups and the mental health community in an attempt to highlight and protest inaccurate portrayals and stigmatizing content (Pirkis, Blood, Dare, and Holland, 2008), or create media reporting guidelines (Kisely and Denney,

2007). Because journalists may view reporting guidelines as an attempt to censor content and restrain their journalistic freedom, such activities can result in a backlash and unnecessary polarization. A less intrusive approach has been adopted by the Carter Center in the United States, which offers an international fellowship in mental health journalism. The goals of the fellowship program are to increase accurate reporting of mental health issues and decrease inaccurate and stigmatizing content; to help journalists produce high-quality work that is grounded in a thorough understanding of mental health issues; and to develop a cadre of informed print and electronic journalists who will accurately report mental health stories. The expectation is that informed journalists will have an impact on the public's understanding of mental health and mental illness as well as influence their peers to reduce stigmatizing portrayals. Recipients of the fellowship have come from the United States, New Zealand, Romania, and South Africa, and have produced award-winning books, newspaper articles, radio documentaries, and video documentaries in the area of mental health (Carter Center, 2011). In some countries (such as Ireland and the Philippines), journalists are working collaboratively with mental health personnel to develop guidelines for reporting that do not stigmatize people with a mental illness.

The Mental Health Commission of Canada has targeted journalism students to raise their awareness about the role of media in creating and perpetuating negative stereotypes. The Canadian program uses contact-based education with individuals who have had personal experience with a mental illness, and includes a renowned journalist. This approach has resulted in small but statistically significant improvements in aggregated scale scores, with large and statistically significant improvements in specific items dealing with dangerousness and unpredictability. Half of the students surveyed indicated that they thought their participation in the symposium would change the way they would cover stories involving someone with a mental illness (Stuart, Koller, Christie, and Pietrus, 2011).

These examples highlight the importance of working collaboratively with journalists and other media representatives to improve their understanding of the ways that the media perpetuate stigma, the harmful effects such stigma has for people who have a mental illness and their family members, and the importance of responsible reporting.

Occasionally, the entertainment media releases a movie that provides a positive perspective on mental illness. Members of the World Psychiatric Association's Open the Doors programmed in Germany used the release of two movies depicting people with a mental illness, *A Beautiful Mind* and *White Noise*—both movies depicting characters with schizophrenia—to conduct an open public forum. Both movies were aired and followed by a panel discussion.

Panel members included people with schizophrenia, family members, local mental health advocates, and mental health providers. Following the presentation and discussion, 75% of the audience thought that they had gained more understanding, and 80% said they would empathize more with people who had schizophrenia. At the same time, however, expressions of social distance also increased (Gaebel, Bauman, and Zaske, 2005). The vivid examples of symptoms and their effects that were contained in both films may have produced this unexpected effect, providing evidence for the complex relationship between attitudes and behaviors.

CAN COMMUNITY PROJECTS MAKE A POPULATION DIFFERENCE?

Smaller, intensive interventions that target specific groups and are tailored to the culture and practices of these groups are our recommended approach to stigma reduction. The question that remains is whether such activities, if conducted in sufficient amounts, can yield change that is visible at the population level. This is a particularly important question for anti-stigma initiatives that are funded to implement national programs as, often, the only method considered capable of reaching a national audience is one that employs broadbased media strategies. However, as we have demonstrated, media campaigns may not be potent enough to bring about meaningful attitude change, and they may have little or no impact on discriminatory practices or behaviors. If national programs are to be persuaded to adopt a new paradigm based on a community development approach, then they must also be convinced that such an approach will ultimately yield results that are measurable at the population level—and there is some evidence that they can.

Germany initiated a large anti-stigma program in 1999 as part of the World Psychiatric Association's *Open the Doors* global anti-stigma program (Gaebel et al., 2008). Between 2001 (when the program was fully operational) and 2004, various local anti-stigma interventions were undertaken, all of which emphasized contact-based education. These included lectures at adult education centers, art exhibitions, cinema events, readings, theatre events, and charity concerts. Most events included panel discussions with mental health professionals and people who had experienced a mental illness. Press conferences were held prior to the events, and press workshops were held to improve media reporting. Selected interventions were evaluated and consistently showed positive results. However, the effectiveness of these interventions and the resulting media reports about them bringing about change at the population level remained open to question. To address this question, the evaluation team conducted representative surveys in 2001 and 2004 in locations with and without the anti-stigma programs. The samples were representative, had a high initial response rate (75%), and a good follow-up rate (64%). Two locations (Dusseldorf and Munich) had received the *Open the Doors* anti-stigma programming. Two locations (Cologne and Bonn) had received awareness programs to enhance early recognition of schizophrenia, which were targeted to teachers and general practitioners. Two locations (Berlin and Essen) were control sites, neither having anti-stigma nor awareness programs.

Results showed that small, statistically significant differences in social distance scores occurred in Dusseldorf and Munich—the sites of the anti-stigma programming—but not in any of the other locations. Although public knowledge of the anti-stigma interventions was low (6.7%), those who knew of one of the anti-stigma initiatives showed a higher-than-average decrease in social distance scores. These were also respondents who were more likely to report knowing someone with a mental illness (8.4% of those who knew of an anti-stigma program, compared to 4.4% of those who did not). Most of the knowledge variables were not significantly correlated with drops in social distance, with two exceptions. People who supported outpatient treatment were less socially distancing, and those who thought that people with schizophrenia were dangerous were more socially distancing. Though social distance measures are considered to be predictive of behavior, they are not direct measures, so it is unclear whether these results would correspond to changes in the personal experiences of people who have a mental illness. Nevertheless, these results support the view that locally targeted and conducted anti-stigma programs can exert population effects. To our knowledge, this is the first study that has examined the effects of local anti-stigma efforts at a population level using a repeated measures design.

In 2009, the Mental Health Commission of Canada launched a national anti-stigma initiative entitled *Opening Minds*. This program is working with grass-roots organizations, through formal partnerships, to develop best practices in anti-stigma programming targeted to youth, health providers, workplaces, and the media. Activities center on creating structural change at the level of organizational structures and processes, and incorporating contact-based components into existing anti-stigma efforts. More than 50 pilot projects have been identified, most of which are actively developing and testing program materials. As best practices are developed, public awareness activities will be employed to encourage uptake of these resources. A unique feature of this program is the deliberate development of knowledge networks wherein the program acts as a catalyst to mobilize and focus the actions of others to make a difference in the lives of people who have a mental illness (Mental Health Commission of Canada, 2011).

As these selected examples illustrate, fighting stigma and discrimination is an important public health goal that is gaining stature. Smaller, focused anti-stigma programs that employ promising practices (such as contact-based active education) may be more effective in bringing about meaningful change. While research is still preliminary, and much remains to be learned, these programs have shown considerable promise. Moreover, they challenge the notion that stigma is so entrenched that no program can ever prevent or reduce it.

13

Summary of Part I

There is no doubt that the stigma attached to mental illnesses casts a long shadow. Not only does it affect those who have a mental illness, it undermines both social and professional support systems. Stigma denigrates the value of people who have a mental illness, and it maintains mental health programs and systems at low levels of priority for government funders. It reduces the quality of life of people who have a mental illness and that of their family members, and creates inequities in the quality and availability of treatments.

Stigma is attached to mental illness in most parts of the world; however, religion and culture influence the nature and consequences of stigma. In developed countries, consideration of what constitutes a minimally acceptable quality of life is inextricably tied to the notion of having a home, a job, and a friend. Yet, in the post-deinstitutionalization era, not having these things has become the hallmark of having a mental illnesses. Despite highly advanced legislative and policy frameworks, developed countries have not eliminated prejudice and discrimination related to mental illness. So far, second-generation protections (emphasizing social entitlements) have been unsuccessful in eliminating systemic discrimination experienced by people with a mental illness who find themselves caught in a tetrad of misfortunes based on poverty, disenfranchisement, powerlessness, and championlessness (Callard et al., 2011).

Stigma manifests itself in different ways in different cultures. In cultures that emphasize collectivism over individualism, highly disorganized and disruptive behaviors, which result in danger to the self or others and interfere with social functioning, are the subject of considerable shame and embarrassment. In cultures with strong familial ties and traditional values, mental illnesses may bring great shame onto the family and hurt its prospects and development. In these cultures, more-traditional values may give rise to a greater degree of ostracism and social marginalization for people who have a severe mental illness and their families, though less-disruptive forms of mental illness may be viewed with more tolerance.

Because the nature and expression of stigma varies according to local contexts, anti-stigma activities also must be locally grounded and carefully targeted to build on religious, moral, and social frameworks. One size will not fit all. This also means that any country—small or large, rich or poor, industrialized or developing—can undertake credible anti-stigma activities. The pervasiveness of stigma affords multiple opportunities and points of intervention for anti-stigma programming; at system-wide, organizational, interpersonal, and individual levels. In addition to programs that target individual behaviors, anti-stigma programs must also address structural inequities through more forceful translation of existing laws into policies and practices at broad social and organizational levels. Eradicating systemic discrimination through structural change must become an important priority for anti-stigma advocates and program planners. Multipronged programs, which are coordinated across levels, will be a powerful anti-stigma strategy.

Given multiple points of departure, the best way to target an anti-stigma program is to seek to understand the real-life experiences of individuals who experience stigma. Understanding their lived experiences will help anti-stigma programmers develop a more fine-grained understanding of the multiple intersecting forces that produce inequities for people with a mental illness, as well as the most useful points of intervention—points of intervention that are grounded in the understanding that they have the potential to make a real difference in the day-to-day lives of people who are stigmatized. Moving beyond a qualitative understanding of stigma and toward an epidemiology of personal stigma experiences and their impact will ultimately aid anti-stigma programmers by helping them target programs to the areas of highest need, and monitor change at a population level.

Science is a process of "de-contextualizing" and generalizing beyond local contexts: from the particular to the universal. Science also has to adapt or develop new methodologies that are appropriate for specific situations. We advocate an approach that is pragmatic, decision-oriented, and grounded in the day-to-day experiences of people who have a mental illness. Program targets need to resonate with local stakeholders and be chosen strategically, if they are to provide opportunities for success. Programs that employ networks of interested stakeholders and collaborators provide a robust and sustainable approach to local anti-stigma programming that maximizes local interest and expertise. Top-down approaches to the development of anti-stigma targets and large-scale, bureaucratically based programs will not be as responsive to local needs or flexible enough to take advantage of important opportunities as they emerge. Simple evaluation strategies are recommended to promote program improvement, the development of best practices, and a culture of learning among network partners.

Though the goal of eradicating stigma is a long-term enterprise, long-term, specific plans are not necessary for useful action against stigma. Certain general principles have to be developed and understood, but action against stigma should be guided by "enlightened opportunism," defined as a readiness to use important windows of opportunity that might be a consequence of local political, economic, or other change. Programs combating stigma must be able to use these opportunities in order to create quick wins, which will demonstrate that success is possible, energize action, and provide momentum. The structure that could best facilitate the practice of enlightened opportunism is one that is locally grounded (bottom-up, rather than top-down) and builds on multi-agency partnerships in order to create networks of practice.

Mental health professionals and organizations have come late to the advocacy arena and are undermined in their effectiveness because of their dual role as therapists and agents of social control, and their tendency to give double messages about violence and unpredictability. Consequently, mental health professionals should not assume that they will be welcomed into leadership positions in anti-stigma efforts, or that they will garner any credibility because of their professional knowledge, when it comes to community-based anti-stigma programs. Professional expertise does not equip them with the knowledge and skills needed to lead anti-stigma programs. What is more, mental health professionals are often not aware of the various facets of their own behavior that add to the stigmatization and marginalization of people who have a mental illness. Successful leadership of anti-stigma programs depends on personality traits, previous advocacy experience, and a thorough knowledge about the area in which the program will be delivered, more than on professional education. Psychiatrists and other mental health professionals would do better to support community anti-stigma activities by developing strong and supportive partnerships with existing family and advocacy groups rather than taking the reins. They must also come to recognize that they themselves are important targets for anti-stigma activities.

In choosing anti-stigma targets, it is important to remember that small improvements in knowledge or attitudes will probably not translate into important improvements in the life chances of people who have a mental illness. Mental health literacy programs are best suited to improving knowledge and promoting greater recognition, detection, and management of mental health problems. The extent to which they may also improve prejudicial attitudes and reduce discriminatory behaviors is, at best, equivocal, and, at worst, paradoxical. Greater "medical" knowledge about the symptoms, causes, and consequences of mental illnesses can entrench social divisions, particularly for more serious conditions. Therefore, programmers should not assume that improving knowledge about mental illness will reduce stigma and discrimination. Similarly, programs that exclusively focus on attitude change are missing an important opportunity to improve the day-to-day experiences of people who live with a mental disorder and their family members—so much so that we would argue that an anti-stigma program that only changes public attitudes cannot be considered successful. Moreover, the lack of concordance between attitudes and discriminatory behaviors means that longer-term behavioral change cannot be assumed. If the ultimate goal is to improve the life chances of people who have a mental illness, anti-stigma programs must directly target the behaviors, the social structures, and the power relationships that erect barriers to their full and effective social participation.

Despite the popular view that campaigns against stigma are an excellent way of reducing the stigma and discrimination associated with mental illness, and the knee-jerk impulse to mount a large and generic media blitz as the first salvo in any anti-stigma program, media messages may be better viewed as a dubious investment that does not have strong supporting evidence. At best, media campaigns are a blunt instrument. They cannot be targeted to meet local conditions; they are confined to broad generic messages; they do little to alter social and structural forces that entrench discrimination; and they are costly to implement and evaluate. They are better suited to marketing commodities than social inclusion. The situation may be different if media campaigns are embedded in and harmonious with comprehensive anti-stigma programs.

In their attempt to mainstream mental illnesses, many anti-stigma advocates have disseminated the message that mental illnesses are just like any other illnesses—meaning that they have genetic and biological causes that are understandable and treatable within a medical framework. Biological explanations for mental illnesses, however, reinforce the public's perceptions of dangerousness, uncontrollability, and untreatability, and so increase public concern, desire for social distance, and support for coercive interventions. Therefore, anti-stigma programs may do well to avoid seating mental illnesses within any causal or etiological framework in favor of focusing on social and political barriers to social inclusion. Anti-stigma programs should not be built on the premise that mental illnesses are illnesses like any other. Historical and political processes have rendered them different, and these realities must be acknowledged in order to overcome the discrimination and social exclusion that people with mental illnesses face.

Many countries still rely on large, custodial institutions. Shifting the locus of mental health care from large mental hospitals to community-based alternatives is not an automatic fix for stigma. Communities are often ill prepared to accept and include people with a mental illness into mainstream life. Targeted stigma-reduction efforts are needed in advance of deinstitutionalization in order to insure that people with mental illnesses have appropriate access to physical and mental health services and supports, and that the professionals providing these supports and services do so in a manner that promotes recovery-oriented care.

IMPLICATIONS FOR ANTI-STIGMA PROGRAMMING—PARADIGMS LOST

The implications of this perspective for anti-stigma programming are summarized in Table 13-1. In the old paradigm, stigma was believed to stem from ignorance and misinformation about the prevalence and nature of mental illnesses. Stigma was considered to be a generic social process that applied to "mental illness," suggesting a homogeneous group of individuals, all of whom have similar illness-related characteristics and are treated in socially similar ways. In the new paradigm, stigma is conceptualized as evolving along various

Table 13-1. IMPLICATIONS FOR ANTI-STIGMA PROGRAMMING

Program Components	Paradigm Lost	New Paradigm
Origins of stigma	Stigma is a result of Ignorance and misinformation.	Stigma occurs at multiple reinforcing levels; individual, interpersonal, and structural
The nature of stigma	Stigma is generic and homogeneous across large populations	Stigma is culturally specific, locally applied, and differs depending on the mental condition considered
Selection of program objectives	On the basis of scientific evidence	Discussions with people who have a mental illness and their relatives
Targets of anti-stigma activities	The general population	Sharply defined groups within the population
Scope of programs	Large, social marketing projects with considerable external funding	Small, locally situated programs and networks of programs that manage with modest budgets and considerable volunteer support
Duration of the program	Campaigns of short duration, say up to 3 to 5 years	Anti-stigma programs that are sustainable and incorporated as a routine part of activities

(continued)

Table 13-1. (CONTINUED)

Program Components	Paradigm Lost	New Paradigm
Overarching goals	Improved knowledge and attitudes	Improved life chances for and social inclusion of people who have a mental illness; removal of social and structural barriers to full and effective social participation
Benchmarks of success	Improved self-reported knowledge and attitudes	Changes in discriminatory behaviors and structural inequities
Role of people with a mental illness	Recipients and beneficiaries of anti-stigma programs	Active participants and leaders of programs
Role of mental health professionals	Purveyors of clinical knowledge and leaders of anti-stigma programs	A target for anti-stigma activities and partners in community-based anti-stigma work.
Legal provisions	Ensure protection against coercion, abuse and loss of freedom (negative rights)	Promote social inclusion through legislation that insures equitable access to housing, employment, and disability supports (positive rights)
Organization of services	Increased accessibility to community-based care will destigmatize people with a mental illness	Recovery-oriented care will help people with a mental illness develop meaning
Educational approach	Factual and didactic, driven by expert knowledge about the biological basis of mental illnesses	Experiential and active, driven by personal recovery stories and personal contact
Program evaluation	Programs not systematically evaluated; assumed that they work	Systematic evaluation of programs in order to create best-practice models

social dimensions that function in mutually reinforcing ways at interpersonal and structural levels. Though stigma is considered to be a global problem, there is greater recognition that stigma plays out in ways that are specific to local contexts and to particular mental illnesses, and that these must be specifically addressed by anti-stigma programs.

In the old paradigm, programs were developed using a top-down approach, often based on review of the scientific evidence to establish appropriate goals. They were broad in scope, targeting entire populations, and employed social marketing to demythologize mental illnesses with factual information. Funding was typically external (such as from government grants) and budgets were large. Often conceptualized as "campaigns," they involved bursts of media activity which tended to lapse after a brief period (such as three to five years). In the new paradigm, programmers sharply define target groups and employ more tailored interventions. A bottom-up approach is used to define program targets that center on the priorities of people who have a mental illness and their family members. Programs are smaller in scope; they may network to share resources, have modest budgets, and rely heavily on volunteer and in-kind resources, thus making them more sustainable. In the new paradigm, everyone can contribute to anti-stigma programming.

In the old paradigm, the goals of anti-stigma programs were to improve knowledge and attitudes of the general public toward "mental illness" or, in some cases, specific mental illnesses, such as depression or schizophrenia. The assumption was that improved knowledge would eventually, over the long run, translate into improved attitudes, which in turn, would translate into less discrimination. In the new paradigm, the assumption that improved knowledge and attitudes translate into improved life chances for people with a mental illness and greater social inclusion is not made. Rather, behavioral outcomes are targeted directly, and benchmarks of success are those that indicate reduced discrimination and structural inequities. In the new paradigm, anti-stigma efforts use a model based on experiential and active learning that centers on people who have a mental illness sharing their recovery stories. Positive contact with people who are recovered or recovering from an illness breaks down social barriers and removes much of the discomfort people feel in engaging with people who have a mental illness. Contact-based models are also empowering for the people who deliver the educational interventions, and so provide a win-win situation.

In the old paradigm, people with a mental illness tended to be viewed as the passive recipients or beneficiaries of anti-stigma programs. Factual information was often provided by professionals, who took a leading role in the development of campaign messages as purveyors of clinical knowledge. In the new paradigm, clinical knowledge is considered to be of secondary importance and may even be counterproductive. The active involvement of people with a mental health problem is central to anti-stigma efforts, and professional groups should take on supporting roles: functioning as partners in community-based anti-stigma work. The new paradigm also recognizes that the health and mental health professionals are important targets for anti-stigma interventions owing to their own prejudicial attitudes and discriminatory behaviors.

In the old paradigm, legal provisions concentrated on protecting people with a mental illness against arbitrary detention, coercive treatment, and other infringements on their personal freedoms. In the new paradigm, such first-generation protections have evolved into legal and policy supports for positive rights that are designed to insure equitable access to housing, employment, and disability supports in order to foster full and effective social participation for all disabled people. The organization of mental health services has similarly evolved, from a model that emphasizes the deinstitutionalization of large and custodial mental hospitals (still common in many parts of the world) to community-based alternatives: services and supports that promote independent living and recovery. In this context, recovery is conceptualized as a personal and transformative journey in which the individual transcends their mental illness as the central and defining feature of their life. In recovery-oriented services, mental health providers work as partners in this process.

In the old paradigm, programs were assumed to work, so they were rarely systematically evaluated. Any evaluations that were conducted were not completed by arms-length groups and seldom found their way into the scientific literature where they could contribute to best-practice guidelines. Programs in the new paradigm take a self-critical perspective and engage in ongoing systematic evaluation. They may work in partnership with local university researchers to ensure evaluation models that meet scientific standards for rigor and objectivity and make sure the results will contribute to the legacy of best practice literature.

Finally, in the new paradigm, much can be done by "regular" people in the interests of reducing stigma attributed to mental illnesses. Anti-stigma programs do not have to be nationally coordinated, expensive, or situated in complicated organizational structures. A community development perspective promotes grassroots activities and practice networks that build on local energies and resources as a cost-efficient alternative.

Building Programs Against Stigma and Its Consequences

Part II is a non-technical training resource designed to help local groups through the process of setting up an anti-stigma program. It draws on our experiences working with international, national, and local anti-stigma groups and is intended to serve as a "how-to" companion to the theoretical material supplied in Part I. Materials in this section are based on a training manual used by faculty in the *Open the Doors* program to assist individuals with setting up local anti-stigma programs. It has been developed with broad international input (World Psychiatric Association Global Program to Reduce Stigma and Discrimination Because of Schizophrenia, 2005).

14

Getting Going

INTRODUCTION

Many local community groups and coalitions are interested in creating anti-stigma activities in their communities; often with limited resources and largely volunteer labor. This section is targeted to local groups and individuals who wish to conduct an anti-stigma program and provides direction on how to conduct meaningful activities on a limited budget. Advice is pragmatic and based on our experiences with local, national, and international anti-stigma efforts, but particularly with the World Psychiatric Association's global anti-stigma network. These experiences have taught us that everyone can take part in anti-stigma programming, and that modest efforts are possible for anyone to achieve.

DEVELOPING A PROGRAM COMMITTEE

Anti-stigma programs often begin with a small number of interested people, or a small group, who will provide the leadership and the time needed to launch the program. These initial organizers will need a larger group of people to carry out the program's activities. Thus, one of their first tasks will be to develop the program's structure. Often, in a small program, this will involve creating a single action group, or *program committee*, that will oversee and conduct all of the program's activities. In a larger program, multiple task-oriented groups may be established. Figure 14.1 lists potential program and advisory group members.

The composition of the program committee is particularly important, as much of the day-to-day work will be performed by program committee members. Because much of the work will be carried out by volunteers, members must be committed to the goals of the program and willing to devote a substantial amount of time and effort to achieve them.

The size of the program committee is also an important decision. If it is too small, then its members may become tired and burned out. If it is too large,

Individuals with lived experience of a mental illness:
- People who have received treatment
- Family members (parents and children)
- Peer support workers

Opinion leaders:
- Politicians
- Senior members of the Police
- Members of the Clergy
- Members of the local Chamber of Commerce
- Members of local School Boards or Principals
- Local media personalities
- Government officials
- Agency directors
- Public health officials

Individuals with specialized skills:
- Accountants
- Fund raisers
- Mental health experts and researchers
- Librarians
- Researchers
- Teachers
- Doctors
- Advocates
- Lawyers
- Urban planners
- Public relations expert

Figure 14.1 Potential program and advisory members.

then meetings will be unwieldy and the amount of work required of any individual member may be insufficient to cement their commitment to the group. Any more than six to eight people will require a hierarchical structure involving sub-groups that are task-oriented and answer to a smaller steering committee.

With respect to membership, it is important that the program committee have direct access to the expertise required to plan and deliver the program. In particular, this would include a chairperson with good leadership skills and, if possible, community prominence; people with personal experiences of a mental disorder; knowledgeable representatives of the groups that will be targeted by the program; people in community agencies who may be working in the area and have an interest in stigma reduction; a media or communications expert; a financial expert; and an evaluator.

Program groups will need to be *task-oriented*. This means that specific tasks should be assigned to group members and monitored at committee meetings to ensure that they have been completed successfully. Regular meetings will ensure that committee members remain on track and meet program goals. Each successful milestone should be recognized and communicated broadly. Progress reports, newsletters, and web pages are excellent ways to keep people abreast of accomplishments. When tasks have not been accomplished, then the committee must consider the barriers, identify whether it is possible to elim-inate them, or choose a different strategy. Understanding why things do not work is as important as understanding why they do.

Program committee members must follow through on program assignments and report on their activities to the group. Regular meeting attendance is impor-tant for the smooth functioning of the program. It also demonstrates commitment to the group's goals. In order that assigned tasks be clearly communicated, pro-gram committee members should request that minutes or action lists be sent out to all group members immediately following meetings. This will ensure everyone knows what they have agreed to do, and will provide sufficient time to accomplish assigned tasks. Waiting until just before the meeting to send out minutes and reminders will not give people enough lead time to complete their jobs.

CREATING AN ADVISORY COMMITTEE

All programs will benefit from an advisory group—individuals who provide input into program activities and help to provide visibility and political support for program activities. The function of the Advisory Committee is to serve as a political sounding board for program activities, develop good will in the com-munity, and provide technical advice. In setting up advisory groups, program developers should consider including the following:

- Individuals with lived experience of a mental disorder either through personal or family experiences: Their experiences with mental disorders and their experiences with various social and community support systems will be invaluable in helping the program develop goals and objectives that are relevant and meaningful. Every program should have this expertise.
- Individuals who are in positions of power, either within the organization in which the program will take place, or in the broader community: These individuals will be in a position to make decisions

on behalf of their work unit or agency, including committing
resources, such as freeing up staff time to assist with program activities.
- Individuals who are opinion leaders who can command respect, provide
the broader political support for the program, and give credibility to
the project: These may include influential community personalities,
members of important groups and societies, and business leaders.
- Individuals who have technical expertise that the program may require
in order to conduct activities: This may include individuals with:
financial and accounting skills (to organize and manage budgets);
media or communication skills (to assist with public announcements);
research or evaluation expertise (to assist with literature reviews and
program evaluations); and individuals with public relations skills (to
help in developing press releases, setting up press conferences, and
organizing community events); and, of course, mental health experts.

In recruiting individuals for advisory roles, it is important to be specific
about the program's requirements and timelines, the nature of their involvement with the program, and the time commitment and activities required of
advisory group members. Potential advisors must understand the amount of
work involved and the expectations surrounding their specific role so that they
can make a considered decision concerning their involvement.

SETTING CLEAR GOALS

Stigma is a word that is used to refer to various problems, ranging from a lack of
knowledge about the signs and symptoms of common mental disorders, to the
unfair and discriminatory treatment experienced by people who have a mental
disorder. It has also been used in the context of "self-stigma" to define an individual's own reaction to having been diagnosed with a mental disorder as well
as to the negative opinions and social exclusion that may be conferred upon
others, such as family members or friends, who may be close to someone with a
mental disorder. Finally, the term has also been used to refer to the entrenched
inequities that surround service delivery systems that provide care and support
for people who have a mental disorder. Because each one of these outcomes
may entail different activities, it is important to set clear goals that the program
will address. Figure 14.2 lists some of the goals that have been considered under
the broad umbrella of "anti-stigma" work. Identifying which of these (or other)
goals a program will tackle is a key decision that must be made early in the
process; for every other program activity will flow from this. In Part I, we have
argued that goals should be behaviorally oriented and focus on reducing unfair

treatment and social inequities, rather than on knowledge or attitude change. The goals in Figure 14.2 have been selected by groups undertaking anti-stigma programs. Clearly, some of these goals do not correspond to the requirements of the new paradigm of anti-stigma work outlined in Part I.

In conducting a program, these goals would need to be made into more specific and measurable objectives. Thus, for example, when speaking about employment, it would be useful to consider the objective to be "Increasing the numbers of people with mental illnesses who are employed by 20%," or when speaking about health care, say, "Achieve reimbursement parity for mental health care interventions."

CREATING INTEREST

Because awareness about the importance of mental health is increasing, and more people are willing to talk about their personal experiences, many people in the community will understand and support the importance of reducing stigma. Their interest can be harnessed by describing the ways in which the stigma of mental illness can:

- Deter people from seeking professional advice;
- Increase the disability associated with mental disorders;

---

1. Increase awareness of the importance of mental health
2. Increase knowledge of signs and symptoms
3. Increase help seeking (decrease label avoidance)
4. Reduce negative and prejudicial attitudes
5. Increase social tolerance
6. Decrease social distance
7. Increase social participation
8. Reduce discriminatory behaviours
9. Reduce self-stigma (internalized stereotypes)
10. Improve physical structures and housing for people with a mental illness
11. Create advocacy structures
12. Improve funding
13. Improve access to education
14. Improve access to employment
15. Improve quality of care
16. Improve social and health policies

Figure 14.2 Anti-stigma and related goals selected by local programs.

- Negatively impact family functioning and family support;
- Diminish the quality of life for people with a mental disorder and their family members; and
- Infringe on the human rights of people with a mental disorder.

Enthusiasm for a local program can be significantly heightened by associations with larger national or international efforts. As there are many of these ongoing, local programmers should identify prominent anti-stigma efforts and develop associations with them. Interest can also be generated by holding large benefit functions, such as gala dinners or concerts where widely known public personalities participate. Prominent people are increasingly disclosing the fact that they, or members of their families, have had a mental disorder, and many are willing to lend their support to local activities. Press conferences and features on local community television channels are another way of attracting interest for program activities. Finally, it is important not to forget the power of new social media (such as Facebook or Twitter) in reaching audiences, particularly younger people.

Programs do not survive if they do not meet the common interests of their members and partners, or if the program does not bring tangible benefits to all of its members. Thus, it is important to explore potential stakeholder interests thoroughly before finalizing program structures and goals.

ACQUIRING AND MONITORING RESOURCES

Perhaps the single greatest challenge for local anti-stigma programs is acquiring sufficient financial and logistical resources to maintain activities over a long period of time. The programs that have sustainable program structures and steady funding are the most likely to create permanent change. This often means working within existing agencies and organizations to insure that anti-stigma work becomes a regular part of their activities, supported through in-kind staff resources and institutional structures. Programs that are created *de novo* and are not embedded in regular agency or organizational activities have difficulty maintaining activities and may eventually flounder. An example of a national program that has used a networking model to coordinate activities and build resources is contained in Box 14.1.

Early in the development of the program, the program committee members should evaluate which components of the program will require resources and begin looking for ongoing support for these elements. Many community programs have anti-stigma activities as part of their mandate, and most health care organizations include promoting recovery and quality of care among their

Box 14.1

Working with Existing Programs to Coordinate Activities

As part of its ten-year mandate, the Mental Health Commission of Canada has embarked on an anti-stigma initiative called *Opening Minds* to change the attitudes and behaviors of Canadians toward people with a mental illness. *Opening Minds* takes a targeted approach, focusing on particular groups for change, such as youth or health care providers, and builds on the strengths of existing programs across the country. The program has actively sought out partners and works with local programs to build better practices. Local programs work in broadbased evaluation and dissemination networks. Working with *Opening Minds* staff and a network of university researchers, programs have harmonized evaluation approaches, adopted standardized instruments, and pooled evaluation data to identify areas of strength and weakness in program delivery. Once the best practices have been identified across the networks, toolkits will be created and disseminated widely. In this way, *Opening Minds* acts as a catalyst, building on existing grassroots developments, bringing these programs together, coordinating their activities, and creating effective, sustainable resources.

goals. Thus, it is often possible to develop partnerships with local programs and organizations to support program activities. Formal agreements between organizations and the program committee to redirect some of their activities to meet the program's anti-stigma goals may be the most important source of sustainable funding.

An agency with recognized financial systems will be an important partner if external funding is obtained. This will ensure program accountability and financial transparency by putting some distance between program members and the accounting mechanisms. Funders may have specific financial reporting requirements that must be met as a condition of funding. Funders might also wish to promote a product or their own image, and it is important to avoid identification of the anti-stigma program with the commercial interests of funders.

Writing a Successful Funding Application

From time to time, anti-stigma programs will be able to identify potential sources of external funding they are eligible for, requiring them to write a funding grant application. In some cases, the full grant will be preceded by a letter of intent or a request for interest. These are brief statements that may follow a predetermined format specified by the potential funder. They provide program planners with an opportunity to persuade a potential funder to invite a more detailed application. To be convincing, the program planners must demonstrate that they:

- Have a clear idea about the use of the funding;
- Can link the intervention back to best-practice approaches or indicate why a novel approach should be tried at this time;
- Understand the requirements and strategic objectives of the funder in terms of funding priorities;
- Outline a reasonable plan for monitoring and evaluation (beyond indicating that evaluation would be done); and
- Can manage the project and the project funding to arrive at a successful outcome.

If a full proposal is invited, then the job becomes one of building on the letter of intent in order to convince potential funders that the program should be funded. This requires a highly polished and persuasive "argument" that your proposed use of the funds is cost-effective, will make an important difference, and that this difference fits with the funder's goals and priorities. You must also convince the potential funder that the program team and partners can do what is planned in an efficient, effective, and fiscally accountable manner. Working with partner agencies with experience in receiving and managing external funding, and having a clearly defined evaluation plan, will help you make this point. Projects that are heavily dependent on yet-to-be developed interventions and approaches are likely to cause some concern.

Make the proposal easy to read by compartmentalizing information under clear headings. The headings and subheadings should be able to tell the story. Avoid wall-to-wall text in order to squeeze every bit of information into whatever page restriction is provided, as this gives the impression that there is no clarity of purpose. If the proposal is appealing in appearance and well structured, it will be easier to read and review, will be easier for a funder to defend, and will convey the impression that the program team is thoughtful and well organized. Characteristics of a good grant request are contained in Box 14.2.

Most funders are inundated with requests and must turn down many strong proposals. If your proposal is turned down, try to determine the reasons. Some funders will provide reviewer comments. In other cases, you may need to speak to a representative from the funding agency directly. Try to determine if a stronger proposal would have been more competitive, where the proposal needs to be improved, and whether a future, improved application would be welcomed.

Box 14.2

CHARACTERISTICS OF A GOOD GRANT REQUEST

A good grant proposal is a well-crafted, logical argument that:

- Your program is addressing an important issue;
- Your approach is based on sound principles;
- Your monitoring plan will highlight problems in time to fix them;
- Your evaluation plan will contribute new knowledge about program effectiveness and steer future work; and
- Your budget is reasonable and in line with funder's possibilities.

CHAPTER SUMMARY AND CHAPTER CHECKLIST

This chapter has reviewed some of the key decisions that must be made early in the development of an anti-stigma program and the actions that must be undertaken in order to get a program off the ground. The importance of careful planning is emphasized. The following key questions are provided to guide program planning:

- ☐ Is there a small group of committed individuals who will provide leadership and the time needed to develop an anti-stigma program plan?
- ☐ Is there sufficient support, information, and participation from people who have lived experience with a mental disorder?
- ☐ Do Program Committee members have the necessary expertise to conduct the program activities?
- ☐ Is there an Advisory Committee with broad representation from key stakeholder groups?
- ☐ Do Program Committee members have a clear idea of the resources required to conduct program activities?
- ☐ Is there a resource plan?
- ☐ Is there a system for regularly monitoring progress?
- ☐ Is there community buy-in for the program or a plan for obtaining it?
- ☐ Is there a plan for sustainability?

15

Identifying Program Priorities

A clear understanding of local conditions—particularly the priorities of people who experience stigma—is required in order to target a program and set meaningful objectives. This chapter discusses selected qualitative and quantitative approaches that can be used to assess local priorities and needs.

IDENTIFYING PROGRAM PRIORITIES THROUGH QUALITATIVE INVESTIGATION

Effective anti-stigma programming must be relevant to the needs of people who are stigmatized. Qualitative methods provide a tool for understanding the needs and experiences of those who are stigmatized, and they are an important source of information for program developers. They produce a rich body of information that is expressed in participants' own words. They allow people to qualify their responses and explain their reasoning in ways that structured quantitative approaches cannot. In addition, they can:

- Empower people who have experienced a mental disorder, and their family members, by acknowledging their "expert" role and by soliciting their advice concerning important program targets;
- Help identify and recruit interested and qualified individuals to undertake program activities;
- Help balance the interests of program planners with the perceived needs of the intended beneficiaries of the program; and
- Help create community buy-in from agencies that are also mandated to meet the needs of people with a mental disorder.

Focus Groups

Focus groups are facilitator-guided discussion groups involving six or eight participants that examine a limited number of issues in depth; not to achieve consensus, but in order to elicit a range of opinions and ideas. The group format is used to stimulate thinking and promote a wide range of contributions. Focus groups are a valuable tool for eliciting perspectives that may be missed by more structured techniques. The in-depth information obtained from focus groups is valuable for targeting anti-stigma programs. In addition, focus groups can be used throughout the life of the program to:

- Generate new ideas and concepts to be used to solve problems and troubleshoot when things do not go as planned;
- Create anti-stigma themes and messages concerning what information the program will provide about its own activities; the process of stigmatization; and how the program will position itself with respect to key topics;
- Identify and create support for program activities by inviting people with expertise and leadership to become part of the program development;
- Monitor program activities among program recipients and broader community stakeholders;
- Develop and refine evaluation instruments by reviewing survey instruments for relevance, meaning, clarity, and logic; and
- Take stock of how the program and the group is doing.

Steps in Conducting a Focus Group

Though they may seem easy to execute, successful focus groups require careful planning and preparation. The following steps are recommended:

1. **Clearly define the question or concept to be examined.** Typically, focus groups will address a limited number of open-ended questions in considerable detail. In developing anti-stigma interventions, it may be important to understand what types of stigma experiences people have had; what stigma experiences have the greatest impact on their recovery and quality of life; and what changes, if they could be made, would have the greatest impact on their quality of life and recovery.

2. **Identify a broad range of group participants.** A thorough needs-assessment will capture the views of many different groups, including people who have received or are currently receiving treatment for a mental illness; people with different diagnoses; family members; and people of different ages, genders, and socio-cultural characteristics. Participants who share similar characteristics will more easily identify with each other and engage in discussion, so it is appropriate to plan separate focus groups for each constituency. The goal is to create homogeneous groups of participants with respect to the key characteristics under investigation. Because of the depth of information acquired in focus groups, you are likely to want to restrict the number of groups to no more than six; however, for specific questions (such as reviewing an evaluation instrument), one may be sufficient. Sometimes it is also useful to convene focus groups of people whose stigmatizing behaviors are the target of change, in order to understand their situation and motivations so that realistic interventions can be planned.

3. **Develop discussion questions and probes.** Once the main issue to be discussed in the group is identified, the next step is to develop several open-ended questions and probes that can be used to assist the facilitator in generating discussion and eliciting a broad range of responses. Questions are not followed in a strict sequence, and probes are only used if the group fails to react, discussion peters out, or the discussion wanders off topic. The goal is to use the questions and probes to seed natural and free-flowing conversation among the group members, ensuring that all members have an opportunity to contribute.

4. **Select and train a facilitator and a co-facilitator.** Selecting the right facilitator is the key to the success of the focus groups, as the facilitator is the main "data-collection tool." As well as selecting a seasoned facilitator, you must also consider the fit between the facilitator and the group. A good focus group facilitator will create an open and tolerant atmosphere where every participant feels free to offer opinions. They will be skillful in phrasing questions, a good listener, and display genuine interest. Having a co-facilitator is also important, as this person will take detailed notes. Even when focus groups are audiotaped, detailed notes are required to fill in gaps on the tape or to help sort out details when several people are speaking at once. The co-facilitator will also help the facilitator generate discussion and pick up on important threads of conversation that the facilitator may have missed.

5. **Establish the groups.** Personal invitations with considerable advance notice are necessary in order to recruit enough participants. Personal

communications should be followed up with a written invitation reiter-ating the purpose of the group, the time and location, the nature of the participation, how the information will be used, how an individual's con-fidentiality will be protected, and whether there will be remuneration for participation. Other ways of confirming the invitation may be used in set-tings where mailing might be a problem. It is useful to expect that some people will not show up for the group and always recruit more people than are necessary (at least double). If in the unlikely event that everyone shows up, the two facilitators can split people into separate groups. Providing support for transportation costs is particularly important to successful recruitment. Locate the focus groups in a central, easily accessed location. When speaking to people who are currently receiving treatment about their stigmatizing experiences, it is best to meet somewhere other than their treatment setting, in a neutral location, so that they will feel comfort-able in disclosing stigma experiences from mental health or other treat-ment providers.

6. **Run the groups.** Arrive early in order to test the equipment, arrange the room, and set up refreshments. The facilitator will start the session with introductions, explaining how members were recruited, the purpose of the project, how results will be used, and how the discussion will be han-dled. In most settings, the facilitator will be required to have individuals sign an informed consent form (see Figure 15.1 for an example). Begin the discussion with a general question and have all members respond. A ques-tion that is designed to elicit common experiences (such as their experi-ences of stigma) is a good starting point. As focus groups are intellectually and emotionally taxing for facilitators, no more than three focus-group sessions per week should be scheduled. This will allow facilitators time to debrief, review their notes, identify themes to explore in the next session, look for improvements, and replenish their energy levels.

Troubleshooting in Focus Groups

It is difficult to anticipate group dynamics, so a number of problems can arise that will need to be addressed during the course of the focus group discussions. For example, the group may have a dominant member with strong opinions who monopolizes the conversation and discourages contributions from the others. They may attempt to force agreement amongst members (which is not the pur-pose of the group), and, at times, may usurp the facilitators' roles. It is impor-tant to be appreciative of this individual's knowledge and defuse the situation

This focus group discussion is part of a needs assessment in preparation for an action programme designed to fight the negative attitudes and unfair treatment experienced by people because of their mental illness. We wish to learn about how people with a mental illness are treated by others and develop concrete ideas on how prejudice and discrimination can be reduced. We would like to learn from your experiences.

We would like to talk with you about your views and suggestions on this topic. With your consent, the information you give as part of the focus group discussion will be recorded. Recordings will be used to help us identify important themes. Data will be treated confidentially and will be used only by research staff. At no time will you be identified individually. At the close of the project tapes will be erased and notes will be anonymous.

Consent

I, [name], I agree to take part in the above focus group in line with the conditions described the confidentiality statement.

I understand that the use of audio tapes will be used for the purposes outlined above.

I understand that I will remain anonymous and will not be identified in any way.

_____   _____
             Signature   Date (yy/mm/dd)

Figure 15.1 Example consent form.

by explaining that others' views are equally important. Facilitators may need to be firm and ask them to wait until it is their turn to speak. Establishing clear ground rules for the discussion at the outset will help in preventing and dealing with this problem.

Particularly when discussing sensitive issues, such as stigma experiences, participants may withhold comments due to a lack of trust. Alternatively, they may tailor their statements in accordance with the perceived expectations of the facilitator, particularly if this person is perceived to be associated with a specific community agency or treatment setting. Locating the focus groups away from service agencies, where participants may be known, and asking for concrete examples, rather than opinions, can reduce this problem.

Sometimes focus group discussions can become heated and people begin to express different views. Two participants may begin a discussion that excludes the other group members, either because they agree or disagree. Working in smaller groups, with the two discussants assigned to the same group, may overcome this problem.

Finally, the topics you want to address may be too abstract for some participants, or may not resonate well with their experiences. This often happens when participants are asked to move beyond describing their experiences to envisioning solutions. Avoid questions that ask respondents to solve problems or to move outside of their realm of experiential knowledge. In the context of anti-stigma program development, it is important to understand what would make a difference to group members' quality of life, but asking for specific program solutions is asking them to move beyond their expertise and is likely to result in suggestions to run a public education campaign. Developing specific program approaches will require the combined expertise of the members of the program and advisory committees. Figure 15.2 provides a checklist of activities that must be undertaken to set up a focus group.

Analysis of Focus Group Data

Focus group data may be analyzed in various ways, depending on the purpose of the investigation. The analysis may be broad, intended to provide an overview of issues, or it may be highly detailed in order to develop process models

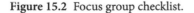

- ▫ Prepare a fact sheet explaining the purpose of the focus group, a confidentiality statement, and a consent form.
- ▫ Invite participants to the focus group at least two weeks in advance of the meeting time.
- ▫ Confirm attendance and give reminders close to the day of the group.
- ▫ Organize technical equipment required (tape recorder, microphone, flip chart, etc.) and conduct pre-tests.
- ▫ Organize the room for the session in a neutral location that is easily accessed.
- ▫ On the day of the focus group post signs showing directions to the room.
- ▫ Bring confidentiality statements and consent forms to the group for signatures.
- ▫ Set up equipment.
- ▫ Organize the seating.
- ▫ Organize refreshments.
- ▫ Welcome participants to the room.

Figure 15.2 Focus group checklist.

or theories. In the case of anti-stigma program planning, an analysis that high-lights the various domains in which stigma is experienced as well as the areas where participants have identified the greatest impact of stigma will be most informative for priority-setting. This can be accomplished by a high-level analysis that identifies general themes and categories contained in the notes. The list of categories that are produced in this way can then be illustrated with verbatim quotes transcribed from the focus group tapes or from verbatim comments collected by the note taker. If high-level themes are all that is required, then it may not be necessary to audiotape the groups.

IDENTIFYING PROGRAM PRIORITIES USING SEMI-STRUCTURED INTERVIEWS

When it is difficult to get the number of people needed for a focus group together in one place, or when you want to protect the confidentiality of people, a semi-structured interview is a good alternative. Semi-structured interviews typically contain a number of questions that the respondent can answer according to fixed response categories, as well as open-ended questions that provide for unstructured, qualitative data. Figure 15.3 provides an example of semi-structured questions that have been used to document the scope and magnitude of stigma experienced by family members. Complete inventories are included in the Appendix and can be used with the permission of the authors. Several translations are also available.

IDENTIFYING PROGRAM PRIORITIES USING SURVEYS

Once problem areas have been identified through qualitative investigation, program committees may consider quantifying their scope and magnitude in potential target groups using a survey. Surveys can provide important baseline data that can be used as a benchmark against which program success may be judged. Survey results are also an important way of raising community consciousness about a problem, which may be preparatory to funding requests. The baseline survey should be conducted prior to implementing program activities in order to insure that the results inform the program plan.

An easy way to conduct a survey is to commission a survey firm that specializes in this area. The advantage of this is that they will have fully developed sampling frames from which to draw samples, trained personnel, and data entry and management capabilities. For example, many survey firms have access to large panels that they have recruited for marketing research. Most external firms will provide a descriptive report and a copy of the data set for

1. Have you felt stigmatized because of your relative's mental illness?

   ▫ Never
   ▫ Rarely
   ▫ Sometimes
   ▫ Often
   ▫ Always

Please Explain:

2. Have other members of your family been stigmatized because of your relative's mental illness?

   ▫ Never
   ▫ Rarely
   ▫ Sometimes
   ▫ Often
   ▫ Always

Please Explain:

3. Could you give us an example of a stigmatizing experience your family has had in the last year?

4. What was the worst experience your family has had?

SOURCE: Stuart H, Koller M, Milev R. (2008) Inventories to Measure the Scope and Impact of Stigma Experiences from the Perspective of Those who are Stigmatized— Consumer and Family. In Arboleda-Flórez J, Sartorius N. (Eds.) *Understanding the Stigma of Mental Illness*. (p. 193-204) London: John Wiley & Sons Ltd.

Figure 15.3 Examples of semi-structured questions asking about family experiences with stigma.

further detailed analysis. In order to ensure that the survey meets the needs of the program committee, members with research experience must work closely with the external survey firm to guide their activities. This may include specifying the target population(s) to be sampled, the nature of the questions to be asked, and the type of analysis to be conducted. Reputable survey firms will also describe a process for pilot-testing and refining survey instruments. This should include a field test on a small number of respondents who are chosen from the target population of interest.

Population surveys can be expensive and may be beyond the budget of many program committees. The cost of a conducting a survey is driven by the number of respondents who need to be accessed and the difficulty of recruiting them. For example, in communities that range in size from 5,000 to 500,000, approximately 400 to 500 respondents will be required to describe their characteristics with a reasonable margin of error (such as plus or minus 3%, 80% of the time). However, larger numbers may be necessary if the ultimate goal is to evaluate change from baseline following program activities, as these changes tend to be small. Program committees should not undertake a survey without access to appropriate expertise.

Several anti-stigma programs worldwide have also worked with national statistical agencies to include relevant questions in their regular survey cycles. This is a cost-effective method of acquiring population-based survey data that ensures regular collection and minimal cost.

There are several things to consider when designing a survey to ensure that the results will be accurate and useful.

- Surveys should have clearly defined objectives and contain questions that are relevant *only* to those objectives. It should be possible to link each question back to a specific objective. This not only ensures that all objectives have been met, but reduces the possibility of gathering extraneous information. Unnecessary data increase the cost of data collection, burden respondents who may refuse to participate if the survey seems too long, and pose challenges for the analysis, which must incorporate and interpret disparate and potentially erroneous data elements.
- For surveys to be used to assess change following the implementation of a program, two identical surveys are required. The first is used to describe the state of affairs before the intervention, and the second describes the state of affairs after the program has been operating for a sufficient period to produce the desired effects. To be comparable, surveys must have identically worded questions, use the same data-collection methods, and target the same sample subjects. If these conditions are met, then the inference that changes observed were a result of the program (not differences in survey design) can be made more forcefully. In addition, it is a good idea to include extra open-ended questions on the post-test to ask respondents whether they benefited from the intervention and in what ways.
- It is important that all surveys be assessed for readability and clarity. Readability statistics can be found in most

word-processing software packages. For the general public, a Grade 9 reading level or less is recommended. Surveys that are intended for schoolchildren should be much lower and appropriate to the grade level being targeted for the program. If respondents cannot understand the questions, then the quality of the data will be compromised. Abstract questions are particularly difficult for younger children and respondents from socially marginalized groups who may be poorly educated.

- Surveys can be administered in a number of ways: face to face, by telephone, with paper and pencil, and via email. Whichever the method, it is important to send introductory notes to eligible respondents to explain the purpose of the survey, how they were selected, and the importance of responding. Follow-up reminder notes can be sent periodically afterwards to improve response rates.

- Survey instruments that have been used by others in similar situations are preferred to those that are developed on the spot. Survey instruments are usually easily obtained by searching the scientific literature—a process that will be greatly facilitated with the assistance of a reference librarian or researcher. Sometimes it is possible to adapt or amalgamate different survey questionnaires to give a more tailored instrument. When adapting questions from other cultures and contexts, it is important to apply the necessary measures to ensure the equivalence of the translated and original versions, and ensure that the survey instrument is acceptable and usable in the new culture. It will also be necessary to pilot-test the instrument (such as in a focus group) in order to make sure that the content is easily understood and applicable to the new context.

- A key challenge for needs assessment and population surveys lies in enumerating all of the people who would be eligible, in order to draw a representative sample. The value of working with external survey firms is that they have detailed enumeration lists that they maintain.

- It is important to keep track of the number of people who do not respond to the survey, so that an accurate response rate can be calculated. This can be difficult in group settings, such as school, when the number of children in class on any given day may not be known to the evaluators. If response rates are unknown or low (under 70%), then findings may be more impeachable and may not warrant publication or broad dissemination. Figure 15.4 gives an example of a letter to participants that can be used in advance of a telephone interview in order to provide information on the study and boost response rates.

Dear Sir or Madam,

Researchers from [Organization name] are conducting a survey of people in [region/country]. The survey will ask for your opinions about mental illnesses and their treatments. This project is funded by [Name funders]. You will be contacted by telephone by an interviewer from [Name of external survey firm] to determine whether or not someone in your household is eligible to participate. Your household was randomly selected from [name source].

Those who are eligible will be invited to participate in an interview that will take about [Interview duration in minutes]. All participants will get a check for [Value of incentive] as token of our appreciation for their time and participation in this important project. Your participation is very important. We want to include the ideas of a wide variety of people, but can only interview people from a limited number of households so your participation is essential.

Participation is completely voluntary. Results will be aggregated statistically so that no individual will be identified. Your responses will remain completely anonymous.

If you have any questions about the research project, please contact [Name of the contact person, position], at [Telephone number] or [Name of the contact person, position], at [Telephone number]. Thank you for considering this opportunity to participate in this important research project. We hope to talk with you soon.

Sincerely,

[Signature, of the person in charge of the project]
[Name of the person in charge of the project, position]

Figure 15.4 Example of a letter to participants sent in advance of telephone interview.

CHAPTER SUMMARY AND CHAPTER CHECKLIST

This chapter has provided an overview of how program priorities may be identified and adapted to local needs using focus groups and in-depth interviews. Both methods share a common strength in providing rich, qualitative information that can be used to understand the nature of stigma experienced by people with a mental illness or their family members. This information can be used by your program committee to develop realistic and relevant targets for program activities will be meaningful to those who are stigmatized. This chapter also discusses the usefulness of survey data with respect to quantifying the scope and magnitude of the problems identified through the qualitative inquiry process. Survey data may be used to build programs aiming to raise community awareness about a problem and attract funding interest. They can also serve as a baseline for future evaluation. The following key activities can be used to guide data collection for purposes of setting program priorities:

- Develop questions and probes that will guide your qualitative needs assessment.
- Identify eligible participants.
- Determine which method (focus group or interview) will work best in your setting.
- Select facilitators (for focus groups) and interviewers (for in-depth interviews).
- Recruit participants and conduct sessions.
- Determine if a population survey is required (and can be afforded).
- Recruit a survey firm from a short list developed from local directories or create a survey team from local expertise.
- Work with the survey team to develop methods and the content of the reports.

16

Program Development

After reviewing the qualitative and quantitative data, the program committee will come to a consensus on the priority areas for action and select target groups, which will be the focus of the program's activities.

PICKING TARGET GROUPS

Target groups must be well defined and specific so that intervention strategies can be matched to their particular needs. Different groups will have different needs. This will become apparent from the qualitative and quantitative assessments that have been completed. In many settings, it will be useful to focus on groups that have frequent contact with people who have a mental illness (or their family members) who behave in stigmatizing ways, as even small improvements in these target groups can make an important difference. These groups include journalists, youth, health professionals, members of community neighborhoods (particularly before locating facilities in their midst), judges, police, and policy makers. In Part I, we argued that members of the general public are too heterogeneous to provide useful primary targets for anti-stigma activities, though they may be considered important secondary targets.

Journalists

Journalists often complain that they do not know whom to contact when they want to write a story about a mental illness. Therefore, it is important to identify and connect with local journalists who regularly cover health stories and provide them with a list of experts who can be contacted to discuss mental health issues. Because most newspaper stories fail to include the perspectives of people with lived experience of a mental illness, it is important that people with lived experience be included on the resource list along with local professionals and other potential advisors. It would be advisable to ensure that individuals included on the list have some media training. Training could be organized as one of the program's activities with the help of your advisory committee members. When speaking to journalists, it is important to have a clear idea of several action-oriented messages about the program.

Having prepackaged material that can be used as background to emerging stories is also helpful, as journalists typically have little time to cover events. This could include information about different disorders and their frequency in the population, myths and facts about mental illnesses, resource materials that could direct people to appropriate community agencies should a mental health crisis occur, and correct terminology to use when referring to people with a mental illness.

Working with journalists can be simplified if a journalist is included on the program's advisory committee. This will facilitate regular communications to the field and help create opportunities for stories that are designed to increase the public's awareness of the issues and how the program is working to address these. Journalists may also help advertise program resources that are available and best-practice approaches.

Youth

Youth are an important strategic target for anti-stigma activities for a number of reasons:

- Most serious mental illnesses begin during adolescence;
- A large number of young people can be accessed in schools;
- Youth are receptive to new experiences and often appreciate having an opportunity to talk openly about mental illnesses;
- Youth are highly receptive to meeting someone with a mental illness and hearing about their path to recovery;
- In addition to classroom-based activities, schools offer a broad scope for companion interventions (such as poster competitions, video competitions, student-led plays, art displays, poetry competitions, etc.)
- In many communities, local public health, mental health, and advocacy groups regularly access schools to talk to students, making it possible to build on these existing programs and activities;
- Working in schools also offers the opportunity to change the teaching curriculum to include mental health–related topics and correct misinformation.

Accessing schools means working through school boards and parent–teacher associations. Because mental illness is still a fearful and taboo subject, school representatives may be hesitant to allow students (particularly younger students) to participate in classroom mental health sessions. Therefore, gaining entrance into schools can be challenging. Having a member of the local school board, a principal, or teacher on your advisory committee can greatly facilitate access to schools.

Health Professionals

People with a mental illness and their family members often consider interactions with health professionals (including mental health professionals) among their most stigmatizing experiences. Because they are in contact with them at a time of crisis and vulnerability, stigmatizing attitudes expressed by health professionals can be particularly devastating. Therefore, health professionals present one of the most strategically located, yet challenging, groups for anti-stigma efforts.

Health professionals are notoriously busy and difficult to approach concerning matters related to the stigma of mental illnesses. Often mental health is not a priority, and patients with mental health issues are experienced as disruptive and difficult to manage. Health professionals often do not realize that they behave in stigmatizing ways. Despite the challenges, it is possible to connect with health professionals in a number of ways:

- By attending regular departmental or agency rounds or academic days; or
- Departmental or agency administrative meetings; or
- Quality assurance committees; or
- During scientific conferences and workshops; or
- Through the scientific and peer-reviewed professional literature; or
- During continuing professional development courses and seminars; or
- During university training (for example, through nursing schools or medical schools); or
- Through professional associations.

In many locations, health organizations conduct regular quality-assurance activities, such as follow-up surveys of clients to assess their satisfaction with services. Getting additional questions on these surveys may be a cost-effective way of raising awareness of the effects of stigma and that a program against stigma is needed.

Members of Community Neighborhoods

Targeted interventions designed to influence the attitudes of small neighborhood groups, conducted before the implementation of a community-based program, can be highly effective in reducing community hostility. Each household can be visited by members of the program staff to provide information and address questions. Establishing a community program without forewarning neighbors is likely to provoke an angry response, even among those who would have initially expressed neutral opinions.

While doorstep discussions are useful, residents will also need more permanent educational material, such as pamphlets, videotapes, or a web page. Public meetings in local community centers or halls may also be useful, but it is important to do these following initial discussions so as not to provoke hostility. Small, vocal groups may highjack the meeting and sway the opinions of otherwise neutral participants. Including members from the local speakers' bureau and residents from other neighborhoods with community facilities can allay fears. In some communities, residents of supporting housing projects have made a special point of helping out their neighbors and projecting a positive community image.

Police

The police are important first-responders in many mental health crises and have considerable discretion in how these are to be handled. Despite the frequency with which police come into contact with people who have a mental illness and their family members, they often have little training and may be misinformed about mental illnesses. For example, they may think that people with a mental illness are prone to act in violent and disruptive ways, so may be more likely to use unnecessary force instead of resolving situations through dialogue. Working with police to ensure that they have sufficient training, crisis-management options, and community support is essential. Interventions targeting police officers should aim to: (1) increase mental health literacy, (2) provide skills that will help them recognize symptoms of mental illnesses, and (3) convey information about ways of reducing stigma (such as by increasing empathy, overcoming negative stereotypes, and reducing punitive behaviors). In addition to factual information on how to access local mental health services, police officers would benefit from training that would allow them to develop behavioral competencies and skills necessary to deal with mental health crises.

Given the high frequency with which police come into contact with people who have a mental health problem, police departments are often highly receptive to training opportunities. Police training should be arranged through a police training department and endorsed by senior officers. Ideally, it should form a compulsory part of the regular training curriculum. The program, which should involve a partnership between community agencies and people who have experienced a mental illness, could help address the mental health needs of officers as well. In working with police, it is important that:

- Senior staff receive mental health training as well as police officers and members of the civilian police force;
- The training programs be based on interaction between officers, members of the mental health community, and people with an experience of mental illness; and
- Tools and materials that are designed to assist police in dealing with mental health crises be provided.

Policy Makers and Legislators

In many parts of the world, mental health legislation is absent or has stagnated. It may contain archaic bylaws, regulations, or stipulations from an earlier, institutional era. In many developing countries, laws may be obsolete (having been introduced in colonial times and not changed since then) or inappropriate for the culture and setting (having been drafted using models from colonizing or highly developed countries). Health-related legislative and policy guidelines often make no mention of "mental health" or make no provision for recovery. Thus the needs of people who have a mental illness such as with respect to employment, social welfare benefits, safe housing, or educational supports, remain among the most neglected policy issues. Mental health advocates and other stakeholders in the mental health community can systematically document inequities and problem areas (such as through program needs-assessment activities) in order to bring them to the attention of policy makers through fact sheets, media reports, press releases, technical reports, and special presentations. Policy makers are highly influenced by what receives attention in the news, so working with journalists can facilitate access to policy arenas.

CHOOSING A PROGRAM APPROACH

Once program objectives and target groups are clear, it is useful to conduct a scan of existing program approaches and their effectiveness. This will require a thoughtful review of published evaluation literature as well as technical reports that may be available on web sites of national programs. Accessing literature exploring possible ways to proceed will be facilitated by including researchers on your program and advisory committees.

The approach you select for program implementation should have demonstrated effectiveness with respect to the program objectives identified. Ideally, it should have been previously applied to the target audience and fit the needs of the target group as identified in the program's qualitative and/or quantitative assessment of needs. It must also be acceptable to them and based on sound logic. For example, if stigmatizing attitudes in health providers are deeply engrained (and, therefore, difficult to change), it is unlikely that a 30-second radio commercial broadcast to the general public would make a difference. What might be more effective would be the development of an in-service, continuing professional education course (or series of courses), that will provide continuing education credits and will be compulsory for all professional staff. In short, the intervention must be appropriate (make sense in light of what is known) and be delivered with sufficient power to make a difference.

Creating a Program Logic Model

Programs are linked sets of activities that are designed to produce some outcome. A *program logic model* defines these various activities and shows how they relate to each other and to the desired program effects to form a causal chain of action. For example, a program that has set a behavioral objective, and then provides only minimal factual information to participants, may have difficulty showing that its conduct will lead to the change of behavior as stated in the program's goals.

The program logic model is the roadmap that links the program's available resources to the program activities, and then to the outcomes that are to be achieved. The logic model spells out how the program produces results, so it is the basic guide for anyone wanting to reproduce the program elsewhere. The process of developing a logic model should occur as part of the program-planning activities. It typically involves a group working together to understand the rationale for the program (in light of needs assessments); how activities will meet these needs; what series of steps need to be implemented to meet objectives; how objectives interrelate to the program's overarching goals; and the conditions under which program success is most likely. It is the theory on which the program rests.

Program logic should be based on the best evidence from the scientific literature, and when this does not exist, on a reasonable set of propositions that can be justified on the basis of common sense. A formal review of the program's logic model can be an important step in the evaluation process. Comparing the logical steps to the actual activities that were implemented can be informative and highlight areas where program effects may be compromised. When there is a clearly articulated chain of events, evaluation activities stand a better chance of improving understanding of what works, under what circumstances, and for whom. Having clearly defined and validated program logic is also important when it comes time to replicate the program in another setting, as it will be important to ensure that the active ingredients are implemented as intended.

Creating a logic model requires clarity of thinking in order to highlight where assumptions may be tenuous or need additional evaluation; where necessary service links are weak; or where elements in the broader environment may impede success. The model becomes a focal point for discussion and consensus, and provides program committee members with an important tool for describing your program to others. Figure 16.1 contains a basic template that may be used to construct a program logic model.

A key component of the logic model is a clear statement of objectives. *Objectives* state the ways in which the program will address the broader goals. Good objectives are:

- Specific
- Prioritized

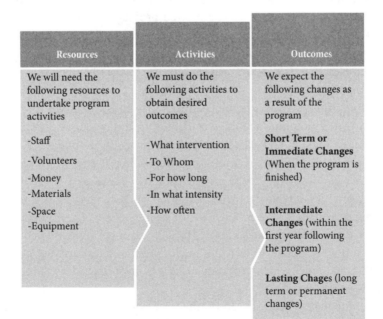

Resources	Activities	Outcomes
We will need the following resources to undertake program activities	We must do the following activities to obtain desired outcomes	We expect the following changes as a result of the program
-Staff	-What intervention	**Short Term or Immediate Changes** (When the program is finished)
-Volunteers	-To Whom	
-Money	-For how long	
-Materials	-In what intensity	
-Space	-How often	**Intermediate Changes** (within the first year following the program)
-Equipment		
		Lasting Chages (long term or permanent changes)

Figure 16.1 Program logic model.

- Feasible, given available resources, personnel, and time
- Measurable, to allow evaluation of the success of the program, such as a percentage change from some baseline level or movement toward some predefined threshold.

If several objectives are set, your program committee members can watch the political, social, and cultural events in the community in order to identify opportunities to create external collaborations. Such collaborations increase the reach of the program, reduce costs, and increase the "buy-in" of community members.

It is important to consider short-term, intermediate, and long-term objectives and how these link together to address program goals. For example, if the goal is to increase social inclusion of people with a mental illness, increasing knowledge or working on attitude change—things that can be accomplished in the short or intermediate term—are not likely to be useful. As shown in Part I, targeting knowledge or attitude improvement does not improve social inclusion for people with a mental illness and may even entrench public expressions of social distance.

A program logic model should contain an *exit clause* describing the conditions that would make it useful and necessary for the program to abandon a particular set of activities and engage in new ones. Similarly, a well-constructed program may be delayed if an opportunity or event emerges that offers an opportunity for a quicker success. A logic model should never constrain a program from capitalizing on these opportunities. It should be a tool that is used to help others understand the program and to communicate program activities, rather than a master of action.

INCLUDING PEOPLE WHO HAVE EXPERIENCED A MENTAL ILLNESS IN PROGRAM DELIVERY

Just as anecdotal stories provided by family members are powerful and important, firsthand stories of people who are living with a mental illness are even more compelling. People with lived experience of a mental illness can discuss symptoms, but more importantly, they can describe the process of recovery and stand in testament to it. They can speak about problems that are relevant to the community group they are addressing, such as what it feels like to receive emergency care when staff members treat you with disrespect; or what it was like in high school when other students teased and bullied them. They can evoke sympathy, understanding, and empathy, and reduce feelings of social distance among audiences.

Therefore, a program, such as a speakers' bureau, that places trained speakers with lived experience of a mental illness into target organizations (schools, police departments, or health settings) can be invaluable. Speaker programs offer an opportunity for collaborations between people who have firsthand experience with a mental illness, their family members, and mental health professionals. Because audiences can become defensive, it is important that speakers be trained to deliver their messages in constructive ways. Advice from educators that may be on the program's advisory committee will be useful.

Public speaking is a stressful event for most people. For people with a mental illness who must retell and relive difficult life experiences, it can be particularly stressful. Therefore, it is important that speakers be protected against burnout that might follow excessive exposure. Burnout can be minimized by:

- Training a number of speakers so that the demand on any one person is not too great;
- Debriefing speakers after events to explore whether they have found the experience stressful and, if so, plan activities accordingly;
- Introducing speakers to the experience gradually; and
- Creating a supportive culture among speakers to ensure that everyone feels free to stand down from a speaking engagement.

A successful speakers' bureau is likely to develop a strong sense of shared mission and mutual respect. This sense of community is valuable for the recovery process and should be nurtured through regular meetings and rehearsals, social events, and celebratory occasions such as common meals, or by formal acknowledgements or prizes.

FAMILIES

Throughout most of the world, families are the principal caregivers for people with a mental illness, but the degree to which families are organized into advocacy groups varies considerably. Many countries do not have the strong family organizations that exist in some countries of Europe, in Canada, Australia, and the United States. Forming a liaison with such groups, where they exist, is an essential step in gaining cooperation and buy-in from families. In some countries, helping families set up such groups has been the focus of anti-stigma efforts.

Family members can provide valuable testimonial evidence that can be used to highlight the nature of stigma in local organizations. Family members are also key participants in focus groups designed to set program priorities. They not only experience stigma directly, but have a close-up view of the challenges faced by their members in managing a mental illnesses. In some situations, they may be more aware of stigmatizing situations than anyone else.

Family members should be included at every level of program functioning. They can provide invaluable personal experiences to help inform program activities. Also, politicians and administrators are more likely to listen to a family member (or organization) than to a health or mental health professional, which makes family members important allies in any anti-stigma programming efforts.

USING MEDIA WISELY

Many anti-stigma programs have used social marketing and media to raise public awareness. In Part I we argued that broad-based social marketing campaigns are not cost-effective and may entrench, rather than eliminate, stigma. Nevertheless, anti-stigma programs will still want to use a variety of media to make the public aware of their activities and advertise their program successes. Media can be more useful in efforts to communicate the nature of the program and ensure that any toolkits or program materials that are generated reach a wide audience, than in changing attitudes and behaviors of populations.

Working with External Media Experts

Public relations experts can be helpful advisors, especially if they have previous experience dealing with delicate topics that are not easily accepted by the community. Often they will have a regular means of contacting journalists and are knowledgeable about how to set up a press release, press conference, or other public event. They will know the best places and times for public meetings and how to advertise them. Journalists pay greater attention to press releases provided by a known media expert. Public relations experts are also knowledgeable about the technical requirements and equipment needed to produce and print materials such as flyers, brochures, or press kits.

Working with Television

Television has a wide spread. Consequently, if it is possible to advertise program activities on television, a wide audience will have been reached. Television interviews are typically short (lasting only a few minutes), and advertising spots are even shorter (thirty seconds to a minute). One challenge is to have a clear message to convey that can be communicated in a short period of time. A useful approach is to try to get messages across in interviews with reporters who will air them during the news at peak viewing hours. Messages can deal with special themes and program activities, such as the launch of the program itself, innovative new activities, or successful milestones reached. As television advertising is often pricey, it will be difficult to sustain it as a main program activity.

Working with Radio

Radio can be an evocative and memorable medium if used creatively, and radio messaging has certain advantages over television, including being the only medium of news and entertainment that can be accessed while driving. Many radio stations offer free messaging for public service activities, sometimes accompanied with personal interviews. Radio stations will often sponsor local community events (such as walks or runs) and actively promote them in the weeks prior to the event. These are cost-effective ways to advertise community activities and draw attention to important program events.

Working with the Arts

In many countries, people who have a mental illness have used the arts as a way of destigmatizing mental illnesses, including art displays, musical productions, theater, cinematic and video productions, and stand-up comedy. The arts are an ancient form of cultural transmission and a means of promoting positive stereotypes. Providing opportunities for people with a mental illness to express themselves creatively through respected public forums has important benefits for their own personal recovery. When presenting artwork produced by people with a mental illness, it is not useful to accompany its presentation by a note that the author has had a mental illness. It is after they achieve fame that they might influence opinion about the creativity and artistic talent of people with mental illnesses.

PILOT TESTING

It is important to pre-test program strategies and materials in smaller target groups before broadening the program's reach. This will ensure that the program is adequate to meet the objectives and the needs of the target group. Programs that target multiple groups will need to adapt materials for each of the groups. Focus groups can be useful for pilot-testing the acceptability and potential impact of program approaches and can yield some surprising results. Figure 16.2 highlights the importance of pilot testing program materials with members of the group that is targeted by the program before distributing them widely.

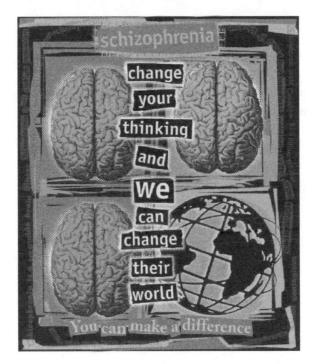

Figure 16.2 Pilot-testing program materials using focus groups: In preparation for a school-based program that included classroom instruction by people with lived experience of a mental illness, a program committee in Canada commissioned a series of posters with reinforcing anti-stigma messages to be placed around the school. The poster art was reviewed by the program committee, and a favorite was chosen. Before putting it into production, focus groups of students were organized. Students unanimously selected the poster (*above*) that the program committee had considered to have the lowest audience appeal. (*Source*: Sartorius, N., and Schulze, H. *Reducing the Stigma of Mental Illness: A Report from a Global Association*. Cambridge University Press, 2005. With permission from Cambridge University Press.)

CHAPTER SUMMARY AND CHAPTER CHECKLIST

In this chapter, we have emphasized the importance of having clearly identified objectives, selecting target groups, then implementing a program that addresses the unique needs of the groups selected. We have briefly summarized key points to consider when working with these groups and have outlined the pros and cons of some of the most popular program approaches and tools. Some of the key target groups identified include: journalists, schools, health professionals, family members, community neighborhoods, police, and policy makers and legislators. The following checklist will help you determine if your program has address all of these key concerns:

- Objectives are based on assessments of local needs that have been systematically examined
- Objectives are specific, prioritized, feasible, and measurable
- Well defined (specific) target groups have been selected
- Program approaches are matched to the needs of the target groups
- People with lived experience of a mental illness and family members are included in the delivery of the program
- Appropriate media have been selected to advertise program activities
- All program materials have been pilot tested among members of the groups targeted

17

Program Monitoring and Evaluation

Program monitoring and evaluation are conducted in order to insure that the program has been implemented as it was intended, and that the expected outcomes are being achieved. The process typically involves the systematic collection of data and a comparison of the actual performance of the program against the amount of change specified in the objectives. Program monitoring and evaluation can uncover both strengths and weaknesses, so considerable effort should be expended to use the results to improve program performance and understand any shortfalls. Program evaluation results can also be invaluable advocacy tools. Successful programs can use their results to create greater policy recognition and attract better funding, and to demonstrate their accountability for funds used. Evaluations may also be used to create new knowledge about best practices in the field of stigma reduction. Consequently, evaluation should be a fundamental component of anti-stigma programming. Box 17.1 lists some of the evaluation questions that may be posed.

Including members with research expertise on your advisory committee will greatly facilitate working with program evaluators to craft an evaluation plan. Evaluators who are external to the program may be perceived as more objective, and their results may hold more sway with funders. In cash-strapped programs, however, evaluation is more often done internally and can promote a culture of critical self-reflection.

Evaluation can best be considered as an iterative cycle, rather than as a specific event that one completes after a program has been implemented. The cycle begins when clear, measurable targets have been defined, and it continues through the life of the program, helping to uncover the logic of the intervention and the short- and long-term impacts. A common mistake is to wait until a program has been implemented before developing evaluation activities—a mistake that can result in lost information and jeopardize the program's ability to demonstrate change. A full evaluation cycle is complete when the results have been presented to the program staff and external stakeholders and used to refine program delivery. Once changes have been made, the process begins anew. By

---

Box 17.1

EXAMPLES OF EVALUATION QUESTIONS TO POSE

- Did the program successfully reach all members of the target group? If not, what portion of the target group was reached?
- How much was invested in terms of time, money, and other resources?
- What was done?
- What happened? Did the program make an important difference in the desired outcome(s)?
- Were there any unanticipated or negative consequences?
- Was the program cost-effective?
- Could the program be successfully replicated elsewhere? If so, what process should be followed?

---

continually monitoring and adjusting activities, programs can ensure that they stay focused; that they do not drift away from original targets; and that their chances of success are maximized. Figure 17.1 describes an evaluation cycle.

USING QUALITATIVE DATA TO MONITOR PROGRAM IMPLEMENTATION

Often the best way to determine what interventions have been delivered by a program and whether they have had any negative or unanticipated consequences is to interview the people who have delivered and received them. Qualitative data are essential to understanding the process and logic of the program as it was delivered, and understanding why something may not have worked. The term "black-box" evaluation refers to the situation in which quantitative data are collected, but cannot be fully interpreted because it is not known how the program actually worked to achieve (or not achieve) change. The techniques of focus group interviews and individual interviewing were discussed in Chapter 15.

ASSESSING CHANGE

Assessing change brought about by an anti-stigma program can be a complex and difficult task. Moreover, the results of any single field-evaluation will never be entirely definitive. Best practices are built on a foundation of many different evaluations being conducted in different settings, with similar (or predictable)

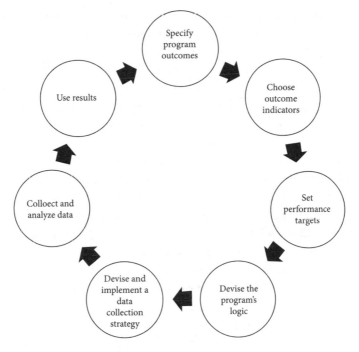

Figure 17.1 The evaluation cycle.

results. Evaluation of change requires at least two data-collection points—one before the intervention and another after the intervention, using the identical instrument both times. Comparing scores before and after then provides some assessment of how much program participants have changed during the course of the program. Additional after-measures may be added to assess how long effects may last. This is a basic, *one group, pre-test post-test design*. It is a useful precursor to more rigorous evaluation approaches and can help determine whether program participants are changing in the expected direction. If not, then more sophisticated designs are contraindicated, as it is not worthwhile to undertake a more expensive and complicated design if the program doesn't seem to be working. If well executed simple designs don't show change, then it is time to rethink the program logic (Posavac, 2011). It is useful to consider a rolling horizon so that planning does not extend too far into the future. In this context, long-term plans do not provide the springboard necessary to take advantage of emerging opportunities. A notion that is of central importance is that well-defined objectives expressed in measurable terms will be the foundation of the evaluation.

In most cases, the application of simple techniques will provide relevant guidance for program planners. It is more important that programs cultivate a culture of critical reflection and inquiry using simple tools, rather than struggle to apply complex analytical techniques that are poorly understood and overly complicated for the job at hand. Simple approaches are more engaging for participants and provide more readily understandable results.

Eventually, more sophisticated data-collection strategies will be needed to more convincingly attribute changes to the program and rule out the potential impact of external events. Inclusion of comparison groups, not exposed to the program, particularly if they are randomly assigned, can help rule out many competing explanations. In the case of mental health–related stigma, the types of external events that could occur might involve a highly sensationalized and publicized act of violence involving someone with a mental illness. Research has shown that such events increase stigma (Angermeyer and Matschinger, 1995). Therefore, if such an event occurs during the delivery of an anti-stigma program, it could wash out or override any program effects, making it appear that the pre- and post-test scores did not change.

Key considerations in assessing program effects are whether people with a mental illness have experienced an improvement in their day-to-day lives and whether they can report fewer stigmatizing experiences. In spite of the fact that most anti-stigma programs exist to improve the experiences of people who have a mental illness, they often fail to measure these changes directly. The challenge is to demonstrate that programs targeting groups such as health providers, youth, or police (for example) bring about noticeable changes in the lives of people who have a mental illness. Figure 17.2 provides an example of a six-item measure that will be used to assess broad population changes over time in people's personal experiences with stigma.

Specification of Program Outcomes

Program outcomes must have strategic importance, be achievable, and be locally relevant. It is important that consensus be reached on these because, unless all stakeholders are working to achieve the same ends, success will be jeopardized. Therefore, the first step in creating a successful evaluation strategy is to clearly articulate the system or behavioral outcomes that the program is supposed to change. The key questions to ask are: "In what ways will program participants (or targets) be different following the program?" "What will change in the environment so that stigma and its consequences are reduced?" Examples of behaviorally oriented outcomes are presented in Figure 17.3.

Social-distance measures have become a mainstay for assessing how members of the public, or subgroups, would feel about socially interacting with people who have a mental illness. Figure 17.4 shows the social distance items that were used to evaluate a radio-based public education campaign that was undertaken

In order to create measure the impact of stigma experiences on people who have a mental illness, Canada's national statistics agency, Statistics Canada, has worked with members of the *Opening Minds* program of the Mental Health Commission of Canada to develop a measure of personal experiences with stigma. The scale will be used to track changes over time at a population level, but could also be used in smaller focussed evaluation efforts. In addition to asking questions about personal contact with people who have had a mental illness, the module asks:

During the past 12 months, did you feel that anyone held negative opinions about you or treated you unfairly because of your past or current emotional or mental health problem? (Yes, No, Don't Know, Refused)

(If yes) Please tell me how this affected you. For each question, answer with a number between 0 and 10; where 0 means you have not been affected while 10 means you have been severely affected.

During the past 12 months, on a scale of 1 to 10, how much did these negative opinions or unfair treatment affect:

...your family relationships?
...your romantic life?
...your work or school life?
...your financial situation?
...your housing situation?
...your health care for physical health problems?

Figure 17.2 Measuring the impact of personal stigma.

- Did important legal or policy change occur?
- Did organizational practices change to be more accommodating for people with a mental illness or their families?
- How many people with a mental illness got a job as a result of program activities?
- Do people with a mental illness and their family members report fewer stigmatizing experiences now that the program has been in operation?
- How many people with a mental illness have gained access to safe and stable housing as a result of the program?
- Do police officers use less force in their interactions with people who have a mental illness who may be exhibiting disturbed behaviour?

Figure 17.3 Examples of behavioral outcomes.

- I would feel ashamed if people knew that someone in my family was diagnosed with schizophrenia
- I would feel afraid to have a conversation with someone who has schizophrenia
- I would be upset or disturbed about working on the same job with someone who has schizophrenia.
- I would be unable to maintain a friendship with someone who has schizophrenia.
- I would feel upset or disturbed about rooming with someone who has schizophrenia.
- I would not marry someone with schizophrenia.

Figure 17.4 Social distance items.

as part of the pilot program for the World Psychiatric Association's global anti-stigma initiative. Items can be scored on a five-point agreement scale ranging from "strongly agree" to "strongly disagree" (Stuart and Arboleda-Flórez, 2001). It is important to keep in mind that social-distance scales measure behavioral intentions expressed in relation to hypothetical situations and may not predict actual behaviors. Surveys of the stigma experiences people who have a mental illness and their family members will provide more definitive evidence that an anti-stigma program has resulted in the desired behavioral changes.

Setting Performance Targets

Once outcomes have been clearly articulated and appropriate measures have been identified, performance targets must be set. Performance targets quantify the amount of change that would be expected to occur for your program to be considered successful. Setting realistic performance targets requires some empirical knowledge. Arbitrarily setting performance targets without some empirical basis can result in problems, particularly if the performance targets are unrealistically high and unachievable. Failure to meet these targets may create a crisis of confidence in the program, among both program staff and external stakeholders. For example, recognizing that it is not easy to eliminate prejudice or discrimination overnight, it may be reasonable to expect a minimum percentage change in scale scores of 5%.

A recent evaluation of a contact-based educational symposium targeting journalism students, for example, reported 5% drop in the average scale score following the intervention, and item-specific changes in the range of 5% to 16% change (Stuart, Koller, Christie, and Pietrus, 2011). An alternate approach was used to set a performance target in an anti-stigma program that targeted high school youth. Rather than comparing average scale scores, an 80% standard of correct answers on the pre- and post-test surveys was used to assess program effect. At baseline, 48% of the students had 80% or more of the items correct. This increased to 79% at post-test, reflecting a statistically significant improvement (Stuart, 2006c).

DEVISING AND IMPLEMENTING A DATA COLLECTION PLAN

The purpose of program evaluation is to reduce uncertainty—in this case, uncertainty about the effectiveness and possible side-effects of an anti-stigma intervention. The importance of having a data collection plan that is feasible cannot be overstated. Complex, overly sophisticated methods, while yielding more scientific and generalizable data, may not be practical for many local programs to implement. Experience shows that starting small, with simple data-collection strategies that gather a minimal amount of data, then working toward more complex investigations as unresolved questions mount, is the strategy that is the most likely to work. Measures that reflect changes experienced by individuals who have a mental illness are preferred to those that measure knowledge and attitudes of program participants, as the former will provide more direct evidence that the program has had an important effect. Multiple sources of data may be required to enable you to fully understand how your program functions, particularly when the goals have involved making legislative or policy changes.

When collecting data, two things are paramount. First, it is important to ensure that all program participants are accounted for, either because they returned an evaluation form, or because they declined. Ideally, 100% of program participants should complete and return usable evaluation forms on both the pre- and the post-test; however, this is rarely the case. It is important that program participants understand that *two* measures will be collected so that they do not miss completing a post-test scale thinking that they have already done one. If program staff do not have direct control over the data collection— such as when a teacher collects data in a classroom—then it is important to provide clear instructions concerning when and how data are to be collected.

Data Management and Analysis

It is important to have access to technical expertise to correctly manage and analyze evaluation data. In many cases, programs collect evaluation data but never manage to marshal the resources to have it entered into a database or analyzed. The highest standard of data quality requires that data be double-entered, compared for mistakes, and then corrected. Findings based on single-entry of data can change substantially when the data are double-entered, owing to mistakes and outliers. Random mistakes in the data may diminish the amount of change detected. When dealing with small changes, as in the case of most anti-stigma programs, poor-quality data can obscure effects. Systematic mistakes made during data entry can reduce or exaggerate results. When double-entering, it is important to have two different people entering the data in order to avoid repeating systematic errors.

Even though data management and analysis may require statistical and technical skills, evaluation reports should be written with lay readers in mind. This means that complicated analyses must be presented in ways that are easily understandable to someone without statistical training. Reports that use technical jargon and short forms are particularly problematic. If results are to be used, they must be understood. Working in partnership with evaluators will enhance the possibility that results will be understood and used. Figure 17.5 outlines the key points to consider when developing a data collection plan.

IDENTIFYING LESSONS LEARNED

Few programs are perfectly good or perfectly bad. If one can learn from mistakes, then the most important contribution of the evaluation is to identify and help explain things that did not go according to plan. Areas where performance was less than expected are just as important to understand as areas where expectations were exceeded. Any unexpected occurrence (good or bad) should be examined closely, given that the overall goal is to identify the "active ingredients" of the program.

Creating a culture of critical self-reflection can be difficult when there are competing pressures to demonstrate that a particular program has "worked." Pilot programs offer a safe haven where mistakes can be made, acknowledged, and studied without fear of retribution. It is often possible, and highly recommended, to implement a pilot phase for the first year of a new program with the expressed goal of undertaking monitoring and preliminary evaluation. In this way, pilot programs can be understood as opportunities to make mistakes and learn from them!

Program evaluations will often provide mixed results. Some aspects of the program will work as intended, and others will encounter difficulties. Having key stakeholders actively involved in the evaluation from the outset will promote

- Instruments and data collection methods should be identical so that any observed changes cannot be explained by the fact that different questions or data collection approaches were used.
- Standardized protocols for collecting and analyzing data ensure that any observed changes are not due to different collection methods.
- Instruments must be able to measure change reliably.
- Instruments must measure what they were intended to measure. This will often mean using an existing instrument with known psychometric properties.
- In addition to being reliable and valid, instruments need to be sensitive enough to detect the kinds of changes that the program is intended to achieve in the time frame allowed and immune to noise from irrelevant questions.
- Instruments should be tested and found to be appropriate in the country and culture in which they are going to be used.
- The measurement window between pre-test and post-test data collection should be sufficient to allow the program effects to materialize, but not so long that they begin to dissipate.
- Data collection procedures must meet ethical standards for research involving human subjects and be reviewed by a local university or other institutional ethics committee.

Figure 17.5 Key Points to Consider When Developing a Data Collection Plan

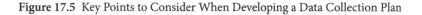

a rich interpretation of mixed results and increase the likelihood that results will be used to make program improvements.

A number of situations can impede the use of evaluation results for quality improvement. Evaluators often look for these challenges in advance and try to mitigate them:

- Funders have explicitly asked for an evaluation in order to determine future funding. Not only will this reduce the willingness of program personnel to be frank about any problems they are having; the opportunity may not exist to make program revisions based on the evaluation results.
- Opposing factions exist within the program and are strongly polarized. In this context, evaluation findings are unlikely to support planned program change and will instead be used to point fingers.
- Political pressures may be such that evaluation findings will be overshadowed by other concerns, as may occur when an unusual

violent incident occurs involving someone with a mental illness during the delivery of the program.
- The evaluation did not incorporate sufficient qualitative data to pinpoint the program processes that should be revised. Consequently, there is insufficient understanding of what accounts for the program outcomes achieved.

ETHICAL ISSUES IN EVALUATION

It is important to be aware of some of the key ethical issues that can arise in an evaluation.

Erroneous Results

People can be hurt by false evaluation findings. Findings that incorrectly show a positive effect, when none existed, are a problem if one considers that the resources used to execute the program could have been used more productively elsewhere. Findings that incorrectly show that a program has no effect, when it does, may result in an alteration or elimination of a beneficial intervention. The latter is a particular risk for a small program, which may not have sufficient resources to achieve a large-enough sample size to detect an important effect.

Getting the right sample size is not only a technical issue, but an ethical one as well. An important determinant of the sample size is the magnitude of the change that can be realistically expected to occur as a result of the program. Large sample sizes are needed in order to detect small differences (which may not be practically important), whereas large differences can be detected in groups that are quite small. If an evaluation is not designed with an understanding of the magnitude of difference that needs to be detected, important changes may be overlooked. Because stigmatizing beliefs and behaviors are well entrenched in the population, anti-stigma evaluations will often require larger sample sizes. If the number of program participants available to be evaluated is too small, then a more qualitative approach should be considered. Technical advice from a researcher will help program planners work through these important decisions.

Anonymity and Confidentiality

People who provide critical information to evaluations may be hurt if their comments are identified or if they can be connected to them. For example, staff members may worry about how their supervisors may react to critical comments about program delivery. People with a mental illness or family members may worry that critical comments will have negative repercussions for their service delivery or access to care. Especially when conducting qualitative interviewing, it is important to ensure that comments cannot be traced back (correctly or incorrectly) to individuals. Similarly, any questionnaire data collected must remain anonymous and confidential.

Given that many evaluation designs require pre-test and post-test measures that must be matched to the same individual, managing confidentiality and anonymity can be challenging. In many situations it will be necessary to create a unique anonymous identifier composed of, for example, the respondent's date of birth, gender, and initials in the first and last names. When working within schools, it may be possible for teachers to assign a unique number to survey instruments and maintain a master list that links the numbers to the students. Conducting unmatched analysis on matched data, particularly when samples are small, can lead to erroneous findings, so matching procedures are an important consideration, with ethical implications.

Withholding an Intervention in Order to Create a Comparison Group

Evaluation designs that use a comparison group that does not receive the program allow for stronger inferences. However, constructing a comparison group may mean that a potentially beneficial intervention is withheld from some individuals. In an organization such as a school, teachers may want all of the students to have access to the program. This issue may be resolved by using a "wait-time" comparison group where "comparison" individuals are put on a waiting list to receive the program at a later date. Alternately, it may be possible to collect data at three points in time—two before the program at different intervals (to act as the comparison condition), and one following the intervention.

Ethics Clearance

Evaluations, particularly those using experimental methods, are not exempt from the ethical considerations outlined in international and national codes of ethical practice for research involving human subjects. In addition, many organizations, such as schools and health facilities, require that formal ethics clearance be received from a university-based ethics committee or comparable alternative. In addition, organizations may have their own internal review and approval process that must be followed before data collection can begin. It is important to be aware of these processes and seek out knowledgeable people within the targeted organizations to help with the application and review process. Creating partnerships with stakeholders who are in the organizations targeted for anti-stigma activities can greatly facilitate this process.

COMMUNICATING RESULTS

There are many different ways of disseminating the results of an anti-stigma program. If the goal is to disseminate best practices in stigma reduction, then two considerations are paramount:

- Evidence-based policy and practice typically begin with a systematic review of the peer-reviewed scientific literature. The strongest evidence comes from studies that show comparable results across different locations and circumstances. Pooled results from multiple randomized trials (termed *meta-analyses*) are often considered to be the gold standard. When experimental evidence (such as from trials) is lacking, then it is important to use replication logic, showing that similar studies conducted under different and challenging circumstance have demonstrated comparable or predictable results. Being able to link the results of programs to the processes that produced them is also important. Unpublished technical reports that summarize the results of evaluations are common, but rarely persuasive. Thus, one important goal is to work with members of the scientific community in order to communicate best practices through regular academic channels.
- In addition to scientific presentations, results must be packaged in such a way that they are relevant for policy audiences. Whereas scientific presentations may be highly technical, policy reports will be more approachable for readers who do not have scientific training or technical expertise. These reports should contain a brief executive summary outlining key findings and recommendations. In addition, policy makers will often prefer a verbal presentation, with time for questions, to a detailed report.

CHAPTER SUMMARY AND CHAPTER CHECKLIST

In this chapter, we have reviewed the importance of evaluating anti-stigma programs and have suggested that this should be approached with an eye to understanding the key active ingredients of the program as well as identifying things that may not have worked as planned. Creating a culture of critical reflection is a key to using evaluation findings to improve program delivery. We have also argued that a combination of qualitative data and quantitative data is important if a rich understanding of program processes and effects is to be achieved. Finally, we have identified the importance of communicating results widely, in the academic literature and through reports and presentations that are relevant to policy audiences. The following checklist outlines the key considerations:

- Does the program have a plan for collecting qualitative data to monitor implementation?
- How will data be collected and used to assess program outcomes?
- Are adequate questionnaires and scales available from the literature?
- What is the plan for pretesting the data collection processes and instruments?
- How will data be managed and analyzed?
- Who will be involved in translating findings into reports that can be understood by lay readers?
- How will the results be used to improve program delivery?
- How will the results be communicated?

BIBLIOGRAPHY AND SUGGESTED READINGS

THE NATURE OF STIGMA

Arboleda-Flórez, J., and Sartorius, N. (eds.). (2008). *Understanding the Stigma of Mental Illness: Theory and Interventions.* West Sussex, England: John Wiley and Sons, Ltd.

Callard, F., Sartorius, N., Arboleda- Flórez, J., Bartlett, P., Helmchen, H., Stuart, H., et al. (2011). *Mental Illness, Discrimination and the Law: Fighting for Social Justice.* London: Wiley-Blackwell.

Corrigan, P. W., Roe, D., and Tsang, H. (2011). *Challenging the Stigma of Mental Illness: Lessons for Therapists and Advocates.* West Sussex, England: John Wiley and Sons, Ltd.

Hinshaw, S. P. (2009). *The Mark of Shame: Stigma of Mental Illness and an Agenda for Change.* Oxford, England: Oxford University Press.

Leff, J., and Warner, R. (2006). *Social Inclusion of People with Mental Illness.* Cambridge, England: Cambridge University Press.

Sartorius, N., and Schulze, H. (2005). *Reducing the Stigma of Mental Illness.* Cambridge, England: Cambridge University Press.

Stuart, H., Arboleda-Flórez, J., and Sartorius, N. (2005). Stigma and Mental Disorders: International Perspectives. *World Psychiatry,* 4 (Supplement 1), 5–62.

Thornicroft, G. (2006). *Shunned. Discrimination Against People with Mental Illness.* Oxford, England: Oxford University Press.

Wahl, O. (1999). *Telling Is Risky Business.* New Brunswick, NJ: Rutgers University Press.

EVALUATION METHODS

Creswell, J. W. (2009). *Research Design. Qualitative, Quantitative and Mixed Methods Approaches* (3rd Ed.) Thousand Oaks, CA: Sage Publications.

Posavac, E. (2011). *Program Evaluation: Methods and Case Studies.* Upper Saddle River, NJ: Prentice Hall.

Rossi, P. H., Lipsey, M. W., and Freeman, H. E. (2004). *Evaluation: A Systematic Approach* (7th Ed.). Thousand Oaks: Sage Publications.

WORKS CITED

Al-Adawi, S., Dorvlo, A., Al-Ismaily, S., Al-Ghafry, D., Al-Noobi, B., Al-Salmi, A., et al. (2002). Perception of and Attitude Towards Mental Illness in Oman. *International Journal of Social Psychiatry,* 48(4), 305–317.

Aldana, L., Miguel, P., and Moreno, L. (2010). The Foundation of the First Western Asylum. *American Journal of Psychiatry, 167*(3), 260.

Allport, G. W. (2000). The Nature of Prejudice. In C. Stangor, *Stereotypes and Prejudice* (pp. 20–48). Philadelphia, PA: Taylor and Francis Group.

Ammam, K. (2005). Situational Analysis: A Framework for Evidence-Based Practice. *School Psychology International, 26*(2), 131–146.

Anderson, R. (1970). The History of Witchcraft: A Review with Some Psychiatric Comments. *The American Journal of Psychiatry, 126*(12), 69–77.

Andreasen, A. R. (2002). Marketing Social Marketing in the Social Change Marketplace. *Journal of Public Policy and Marketing, 21*(1), 3–13.

Angermeyer, M., and Dietrich, S. (2006). Public Beliefs About and Attitudes Towards People with Mental Illness: A Review of Population Studies. *Acta Psychiatrica Scandinavica, 113*, 163–179.

Angermeyer, M., Holzinger, A., and Matschinger, H. (2009). Mental Health Literacy and Attitude Towards People with Mental Illness: A Trend Analysis Based on Population Surveys in the Eastern Part of Germany. *European Psychiatry, 24*, 225–232.

Angermeyer, M., and Matschinger, H. (1995). Violent Attacks on Public Figures by Persons Suffering from Psychiatric Disorders: Their Effect on the Social Distance Toward the Mentally Ill. *European Archives of Psychiatry and Neurosciences, 245*, 159–164.

Anonymous. (2011). News: United States Reviews Safety of Electroconvulsive Therapy. *Canadian Medical Association Journal, 183*(5), E269–E270.

Anonymous. (2011). *TV-Free America*. Retrieved July 16, 2011, from http://www.csun. edu: http://www.csun.edu/science/health/docs/tvandhealth.html.

Arboleda-Flórez, J. (1979). AMOK. *The Bulletin of the American Academy of Psychiatry and the Law, 7*(3), 286–295.

Arboleda-Flórez, J. (2008). The Rights of a Powerless Legion. In J. Arboleda-Flórez and N. Sartorius (eds.), *Understanding the Stigma of Mental Illness: Theory and Interventions* (pp. 1–18). West Sussex, England: John Wiley and Sons Ltd.

Arboleda-Flórez, J. (2011). Psychiatry and the Law: Do the Fields Agree in Their View of Coercive Treatment? In T. W. Kallert, . J. Mezzich, and J. Monahan (eds.), *Coercive Treatment in Psychiatry. Clinical, Legal and Ethical Aspects* (pp. 81–96). Chichester, England: John Wiley and Sons, Ltd.

Arens, D. (1993). What Do the Neighbours Think Now? Community Residences on Long Island, New York. *Community Mental Health Journal, 29*(3), 235–245.

Ayduin, N., Yigit, A., Inandi, T., and Kirpinar, I. (2003). Attitudes of Hospital Staff Toward Mentally Ill Patients in a Teaching Hospital, Turkey. *International Journal of Social Psychiatry, 49*(1), 17–26.

Baker, E., Kan, M., and Teo, S. (2011). Developing a Collaborative Network Organization: Leadership Challenges at Multiple Levels. *Journal of Organizational Change Management, 24*(6), 863–875.

Baker, F., and Douglas, C. (1990). Housing Environments and Community Adjustment of Severely Mentally Ill Persons. *Community Mental Health Journal, 26*(6), 497–505.

Baxter, J., Samnaliev, M., and Clark, R. (2009). The Quality of Asthma Care Among Adults with Substance-Related Disorders and Adults with Mental Illness. *Psychiatric Services, 60*, 43–49.

Beldi, A., den Boer, J., Brain, C., Constant, E., Figueira, M., Filipcic, I., et al. (in press). Fighting Stigma of Mental Illness in Midsize European Countries. *Social Psychiatry and Psychiatric Epidemiology*.

Benbunan-Fich, R., and Hiltz, S. (1999). Impacts of Asynchronous Learning Networks on Individual and Group Problem Solving: A Field Experiment. *Group Decision and Negotiation, 8*, 409–426.

Ben-Zeev, D., Young, M., and Corrigan, P. (2010). *DSM-V* and the Stigma of Mental Illness. *Journal of Mental Health, 19*(4), 318–327.

Black, N. (2001). Evidence Based Policy: Proceed with Care. *British Medical Journal, 323*, 275–279.

Bourget, B., and Chenier, R. (2007). *Mental Health Literacy in Canada: Phase One Draft Report Mental Health Literacy Project*. Ottawa: Canadian Alliance on Mental Illness and Mental Health.

Brohan, E., Elgie, R., Sartorius, N., Thornicroft, G., and GAMIAN-Europe Study Group. (2010). Self-Stigma, Empowerment and Perceived Discrimination Among People with Schizophrenia in 14 European Countries: The GAMIAN-Europe Study. *Schizophrenia Research, 122*, 232–238.

Byrne, P. (2000). Stigma of Mental Illness and Ways of Diminishing It. *Advances in Psychiatric Treatment, 6*, 65–72.

Caldwell, T., and Jorm, A. (2001). Mental Health Nurses' Beliefs About Likely Outcomes for People with Schizophrenia or Depression: A Comparison with the Public and Other Healthcare Professionals. *Australian and New Zealand Journal of Mental Health Nursing, 10*, 42–54.

Callard, F., Sartorius, N., Arboleda-Flórez, J., Bartlett, P., Helmchen, H., Stuart, H., et al. (2011). *Mental Illness, Discrimination and the Law: Fighting for Social Justice*. London: Wiley-Blackwell.

Campbell, C., and Jovchelovitch, S. (2000). Health, Community Development: Towards a Social Psychology of Participation. *Journal of Community and Applied Social Psychology, 10*, 255–270.

Canadian Medical Association. (2008). *Eighth Annual National Report Card on Health Care*. Ottawa: Canadian Medical Association.

Carling, P. (1990). Major Mental Illness, Housing, and Supports. *American Psychologist, 45*(8), 969–975.

Carr, V., Lewin, T., Barnard, R., Walton, J., Allen, J., Constable, P., et al. (2004). Attitudes and Roles of General Practitoners in the Treatment of Schizophrenia Compared with Community Mental Health Staff and Patients. *Social Psychiatry and Psychiatric Epidemiology, 39*, 78–84.

Carr, V., Lewin, T., Walton, J., Faehrmann, C., and Reid, A. (1997). Consultation-Liaison Psychiatry in General Practice. *The Australian and New Zealand Journal of Psychiatry, 31*, 85–94.

Carter Center. (2011). The Rosalynn Carter Fellowships for Mental Health Journalism http://www.cartercenter.org/health/mental_health/fellowships/index.html Retrieved June 17, 2011

Chan, J., Mak, W., and Law, L. (2009). Combining Education and Video-Based Contact to Reduce Stigma of Mental Illness: "The Same or Not the Same" Anti-Stigma Program for Secondary Schools in Hong Kong. *Social Science and Medicine, 68*, 1521–1526.

Charles, H., Manoranjitham, S., and Jacob, K. (2007). Stigma and Explanatory Models Among People with Schizophrenia and Their Relatives in Vellore, South India. *International Journal of Social Psychiatry, 53*(4), 325–332.

Cheung, F. (1990). Brief Program Report: People Against the Mentally Ill: Community Opposition to Residential Treatment Facilities. *Community Mental Health Journal, 26*(2), 205–212.

Chou, K., and Mak, K. (1998). Attitudes to Mental Patients Among Hong Kong Chinese: A Trend Study Over Two Years. *International Journal of Social Psychiatry, 44*(3), 215–224.

Chowdhury, A., Chakraborty, A., and Weiss, M. (2001). Community Mental Health Concepts of Mental Illness in the Sundarban Delta of West Bengal, India. *Anthropology and Medicine, 8*(1), 109–129.

Cobigo, V., and Stuart, H. (2010). Social Inclusion and Mental Health. *Current Opinion in Psychiatry, 23*(5), 453–457.

Coker, E. (2005). Selfhood and Social Distance: Toward a Cultural Understanding of Psychiatric Stigma in Egypt. *Social Science and Medicine, 61*, 920–930.

Cook, J., Leff, H., Blyler, C., Gold, P., Goldberg, R., Mueser, K., et al. (2005). Results of a Multi-site Randomized Trial of Supported Employment Interventions for Individuals with Severe Mental Illness. *Archives of General Psychiatry, 62*, 505–512.

Corrigan, P. W., River, L. P., Lundin, R. K., Penn, D. L., Uphoff-Wasowski, K., Campion, J., et al. (2001). Three Strategies for Changing Attributions About Severe Mental Illness. *Schizophrenia Bulletin, 27*(2), 187–195.

Corrigan, P. W., Roe, D., and Tsang, H. (2011). *Challenging the Stigma of Mental Illness: Lessons for Therapists and Advocates*. West Sussex, England: John Wiley and Sons, Ltd.

Corrigan, P., Markowitz, R., Watson, Q., Rowan, D., and Kubiak, M. (2003). An Attribution Model of Public Discrimination Towards Persons with Mental Illness. *Journal of Health and Social Behavior, 44*(2), 162–179.

Crisp, A. (2000). Changing Minds: Every Family in the Land: An Update on the College's Campaign. *Psychiatric Bulletin, 24*, 267–268.

Crossley, N. (1998). R. D. Laing and the British Anti-Psychiatry Movement: A Socio-Historical Analysis. *Social Science and Medicine, 47*(7), 877–889.

Crowther, R., Marshall, M., Bond, G., and Huxley, P. (2001). Helping People with Severe Mental Illness to Obtain Work: A Systematic Review. *British Medical Journal, 322*, 204–208.

Cumming, E., and Cumming, J. (1957). *Closed Ranks: An Experiment in Mental Health Education*. Cambridge, MA: Harvard University Press.

Dain, N. (1989). Critics and Dissenters: Reflections on "Anti-Psychiatry" in the United States. *Journal of the History of the Behavioural Sciences, 25*, 3–25.

D'Arcy, C. (1987). Opened Ranks? Blackfoot Revisited. In D. Coburn, C. D'Arcy, G. M. Torrence, and P. Newman (eds.), *Health and Canadian Society: Sociological Perspectives* (2nd Ed., pp. 280–294). Richmond Hill, Ontario: Fitzhenry and Whiteside.

Deal, M. (2003). Disabled People's Attitudes Toward Other Impairment Groups: A Hierarchy of Impairments. *Disability and Society, 18*(7), 897–910.

Dear, M. (1992). Understanding and Overcoming the NIMBY Syndrome. *Journal of the American Planning Association, 58*(3), 288–300.

Desai, M., Rosenheck, D. B., and Perlin, J. (2002). Receipt of Nutrition and Exercise Counseling Among Medical Outpatients with Psychiatric and Substance Use Disorders. *Journal of General Internal Medicine, 17*(7), 556–560.

Dewa, C., Lesage, A., Goering, P., and Caveen, M. (2004). Nature and Prevalence of Mental Illness in the Workplace. *HealthcarePapers, 5*(2), 12–25.

Dietrich, A., Beck, M., Bujantugs, B., Kenzine, D., Matschinger, H., and Angermeyer, M. (2004). The Relationship Between Public Causal Beliefs and Social Distance Toward Mentally Ill People. *Australian and New Zealand Journal of Psychiatry, 38*(5), 348–354.

Dmeteo, D., Khasakhala, L., Ongecha-Owuor, F., Kuria, M., Mutiso, V., Syanda, J., et al. (2008). Attitudes Toward Psychiatry: A Survey of Medical Students at the University of Nairobi, Kenya. *Academic Psychiatry, 32*, 154–159.

Doessel, D., Scheurer, R., Chant, D., and Whiteford, H. (2005). Australia's National Mental Health Strategy and Deinstitutionalization: Some Empirical Results. *Australian and New Zealand Journal of Psychiatry, 39*, 989–994.

Dols, M. (1987). Insanity and Its Treatment in Islamic Society. *Medical History, 31*, 1–14.

Druss, B., Bradford, D., Rosenheck, R., Radford, M., and Krumholz, H. (2000). Mental Disorders and Use of Cardiovascular Procedures after Myocardial Infarction. *JAMA, 283*, 506–511.

Druss, B., Bradford, D., Rosenheck, R., Radford, M., and Krumholz, H. (2001). Quality of Medical Care and Excess Mortality in Older Patients with Mental Disorders. *Archives of General Psychiatry, 58*, 565–572.

Eriksson, K., and Westring, C.-G. (1995). Coercive Measures in Psychiatric Care. *Acta Psychiatrica Scandinavica, 92*, 225–230.

European Research Initiative on Community-Based Residential Alternatives for Disabled People. (2003). *Included in Society.* European Commission.

Everett, B. (2004). Best Practices in Workplace Mental Health: An Area for Expanded Research. *HealthcarePapers, 5*(2), 114–116.

Fabrega, H. J. (1991). Psychiatric Stigma in Non-Western Societies. *Comprehensive Psychiatry, 32*(6), 534–551.

Farhall, J., Webster, B., Hocking, B., Leggatt, M., Riess, C., and Young, J. (1998). Training to Enhance Partnerships Between Mental Health Professionals and Family Caregivers: A Comparative Study. *Psychiatric Services, 49*(11), 1488–1490.

Fazel, S., and Danesh, J. (2002). Serious Mental Disorder in 23,000 Prisoners: A Systematic Review of 62 Surveys. *Lancet, 359*, 545–550.

Feifel, D., Moutier, C., and Swerdlow, N. (1999). Attitudes Toward Psychiatry as a Prospective Career Among Students Entering Medical School. *American Journal of Psychiatry, 156*, 1397–1402.

Ferguson, J. E. (2005). Bridging the Gap Between Research and Practice. *Knowledge Management for Development Journal, 1*(3), 46–54.

Florin, P., and Wandersman, A. (1990). An Introduction to Citizen Participation, Voluntary Organizations, and Community Development: Insights for Empowerment Through Research. *American Journal of Community Psychology, 18*(1), 41–54.

Foucault, M. (1975). *Madness and Civilization.* London: Tavistock.

Frayne, S., Halanych, J., Miller, D., Wang, F., Lin, H., Pogach, L., et al. (2005). Disparities in Diabetes Care: Impact of Mental Illness. *Archives of Internal Medicine, 165*, 2631–2638.

Furnham, A., and Chan, E. (2004). Lay Theories of Schizophrenia. A Cross-Cultural Comparison of British and Hong Kong Chinese Attitudes, Attributions and Beliefs. *Social Psychiatry and Psychiatric Epidemiology, 39,* 543–552.

Gabriel, A., and Violato, C. (2010). Depression Literacy Among Patients and the Public: A Literature Review. *Primary Psychiatry, 17*(1), 55–64.

Gaebel, W., Bauman, A., and Zaske, H. (2005). Intervening in a Multi-Level Network: Progress of the German *Open the Doors* Projects. *World Psychiatry, 4*(S1), 16–20.

Gaebel, W., Zaske, H., Baumann, A., Klosterkotter, J., Maier, W., Decker, P., et al. (2008). Evaluation of the German WPA "Program Against Stigma and Discrimination Because of Schizophrenia—Open the Doors." Results from Representative Telephone Surveys Before and After Three Years of Anti-Stigma Interventions. *Schizophrenia Research, 98,* 184–193.

Ganju, V. (2000). The Mental Health System in India. *International Journal of Law and Psychiatry, 23*(3–4), 393–402.

Glover, H. (2005). Recovery Based Service Delivery: Are We Ready to Transform the Words into a Paradigm Shift? *Australian e-Journal for the Advancement of Mental Health, 4*(3), 1–4.

Goffman, E. (1961). *Asylums: Essays on the Social Situation of Mental Patients and Other Inmates.* Garden City, NY: Anchor Books.

Goffman, E. (1963). *Stigma: Notes on the Management of Spoiled Identity.* Englewood Cliffs, NJ: Prentice Hall.

Goodman, R., Speers, M., McLeroy, K., Fawcett, S., Kegler, M., Parker, E., et al. (1998). Identifying and Defining the Dimensions of Community Capacity to Provide a Basis for Measurement. *Health Education and Behaviour, 25*(3), 258–278.

Griffiths, K., Christensen, H., Jorm, A., Evans, K., and Groves, C. (2004). Effect of a Web-based Depression Literacy and Cognitive Behavioural Therapy Interventions on Stigmatising Attitudes to Depression: Randomised Controlled Trial. *British Journal of Psychiatry, 185,* 342–349.

Griffiths, K., Nakane, Y., Christensen, H., Yoshioka, K., Jorm, A., and Nakane, H. (2006). Stigma in Response to Mental Disorders: A Comparison of Australia and Japan. *BMC Psychiatry, 6,* 21.

Guimon, J. (1999). Introduction. In J. Guimon, W. Fischer, and N. Sartorius (eds.), *The Image of Madness.* Basel, Switzerland: Karger.

Hailey, J., and James, R. (2004). "Trees Die From the Top": International Perspectives on NGO Leadership Development. *International Journal of Voluntary and Nonprofit Organizations, 15*(4), 343–353.

Hansen, M., Fink, P., Frydenberg, M., Oxhoj, M., Sondergaard, L., and Munk-Jorgensen, P. (2001). Mental Disorders Among Internal Medical Inpatients. Prevalence, Detection, and Treatment Status. *Journal of Psychosomatic Research, 50,* 199–204.

Haslam, N. (2005). Dimensions of Folk Psychiatry. *Review of General Psychology, 9*(1), 35–47.

Haslam, R., Sayce, N., and Davies, E. (2006). Prejudice and Schizophrenia: A Review of the "Mental Illness Is an Illness Like Any Other" Approach. *Acta Psychiatrica Scandinavica, 114,* 303–318.

Haynes, R. (2002). What Kind of Evidence Is It That Evidence-based Medicine Advocates Want Health Care Providers and Consumers to Pay Attention To? *BMC Health Services Research, 2*(3), 1–7.

Health and Consumer Protection Directorate-General. (2005). Green Paper. Improving the Mental Health of the Population: Towards a Strategy on Mental Health for the European Union. Brussels, Belgium: European Commission.

Henderson, C., and Thornicroft, G. (2009). Stigma and Discrimination in Mental Illness: Time to Change. *The Lancet, 373*, 1928–1930.

Himelhoch, S., Chander, G., Fleishman, J., Hellinger, J., Gaist, P., Gebo, K., et al. (2007). Access to HAART and Utilization of Inpatient Medical Hospital Services Among HIV-Infected Patients with Co-Occurring Serious Mental Illness and Injection Drug Use. *General Hospital Psychiatry, 29*, 518–525.

Hindshaw, S., and Stier, A. (2008). Stigma as Related to Mental Disorders. *Annual Review of Clinical Psychology, 4*, 367–393.

Hopper, K., Harrison, G., Janca, A., and Sartorius, N. (eds.). (2007). *Recovery from Schizophrenia: An International Perspective.* New York: Oxford University Press.

Hugo, M. (2001). Mental Health Professionals' Attitudes Towards People Who Have Experienced a Mental Health Disorder. *Journal of Psychiatric and Mental Health Nursing, 8*, 419–425.

Inandi, T., Aydin, N., Turhan, E., and Gultekin, D. (2008). Social Distance of Medical Students from a Person in a Depression Vignette: A Cross-Sectional Study. *Turkish Journal of Public Health, 6*(1), 19–28.

Jacobson, N., and Curtis, L. (2000). Recovery as Policy in Mental Health Services: Strategies Emerging from the States. *Psychosocial Rehabilitation Journal, 23*(4), 333–341.

Jones, S., Howard, L., and Thornicroft, G. (2008). Diagnositc Overshadowing: Worse Physical Health Care for People with Mental Illness. *Acta Psychiatrica Scandinavica, 118*, 169–171.

Jorm, A. (2000). Mental Health Literacy. *British Journal of Psychiatry, 177*, 396–401.

Jorm, A. F., Christensen, H., and Griffiths, K. M. (2005). The Impact of Beyondblue: The National Depression Initiative on the Australian Public's Recognition of Depression and Beliefs About Treatment. *Australian and New Zealand Journal of Psychiatry, 39*, 248–254.

Jorm, A., Griffiths, K., Christensen, H., Korten, A., Parslow, R., and Rodgers, B. (2003). Providing Information About the Effectiveness of Treatment Options to Depressed People in the Community: A Randomized Controlled Trial of Effects on Mental Health Literacy, Help-Seeking and Symptoms. *Psychological Medicine, 33*, 1071–1079.

Kadri, N. (2005). Schizophrenia and Stigma: A Transcultural Perspective. In A. Okasha and C. Stefanis (eds.), *Perspectives on the Stigma of Mental Illness* (pp. 52–85). Geneva, Switzerland: World Psychiatric Association.

Kadri, N., Manoudi, F., Berrada, S., and Moussaoui, D. (2004). Stigma Impact on Moroccan Families of Patients with Schizophrenia. *Canadian Journal of Psychiatry, 49*, 625–629.

Kapur, R. (1979). The Role of Traditional Healers in Mental Health Care in Rural India. *Social Science and Medicine, 13B*, 24–31.

Kelly, B. (2005). Structural Violence and Schizophrenia. *Social Science and Medicine, 61*, 724–730.

Kesey, K. (1962). *One Flew Over the Cuckoo's Nest.* Toronto: Penguin Books.

Kessler, R., Heeringa, S., Lakoma, M., Petukhova, M., Rupp, A., Schoenbaum, M., et al. (2008). Individual and Societal Effects of Mental Disorders on Earnings in the United States: Results from the National Comorbidity Survey Replication. *American Journal of Psychiatry, 165*, 703–711.

Kisely, A., and Denney, J. (2007). The Portrayal of Suicide and Mental Illness: A Province-Wide Survey in Nova Scotia. *Canadian Journal of Community Mental Health, 26*(1), 113–128.

Kitchener, B., and Jorm, A. (2002). Mental Health First Aid Training for the Public: Evaluation of Effects on Knowledge, Attitudes, and Helping Behavior. *BMC Psychiatry, 2*, 10.

Kohn, R., Saxena, S., Levav, I., and Saraceno, B. (2004). The Treatment Gap in Mental Health Care. *Bulletin of the World Health Organization, 82*, 858–866.

Kramer, H., and Sprenger, J. ([1486] 1971). *Malleus Maleficarum* (M. Summer, trans.). New York: Dover Publications.

Krosnar, K. (2003). Mentally Ill Patients in Central Europe Being Kept in Padlocked, Caged Beds. *British Medical Journal, 29*(327), 1249.

Kurihara, T., Kato, M., Sakamoto, S., Reverger, R., and Kitamura, T. (2000). Public Attitudes Towards the Mentally Ill: A Cross-Cultural Study Between Bali and Tokyo. *Psychiatry and Clinical Neurosciences, 54*, 547–552.

Laing, R. (1965). *The Divided Self: An Existential Study in Sanity and Madness.* Baltimore, MD: Penguin Books.

Lauber, C., Nordt, C., Braunschweig, C., and Rossler, W. (2006). Do Mental Health Proessionals Stigmatize Their Patients? *Acta Psychiatrica Scandinavica, 113*(Suppl. 429), 51–59.

Lee, S. (2002). The Stigma of Schizophrenia: A Transcultural Problem. *Current Opinion in Psychiatry, 15*, 37–41.

Leff, J. (2001). Why Is Care in the Community Perceived as a Failure? *British Journal of Psychiatry, 179*, 381–383.

Leff, J., and Warner, R. (2006). *Social Inclusion of People with Mental Illness.* Cambridge, England: Cambridge University Press.

Levi, L. (2005). Working Life and Mental Health—A Challenge to Psychiatry? *World Psychiatry, 4*(1), 53–57.

Liberman, A. (2000). Networks as Learning Communities. *Journal of Teacher Education, 51*, 221–227.

Liberman, R., and Kopelowicz, A. (2005). Recovery from Schizophrenia: A Concept in Search of Research. *Psychiatric Services, 56*(6), 735–742.

Liimatainen, M., and Gabriel, P. (2000). *Mental Health in the Workplace.* Geneva, Switzerland: International Labour Office.

Link, B. G., and Phelan, J. C. (2001). Conceptualizing Stigma. *Annual Review of Sociology, 27*, 363–385.

Link, B., and Cullen, F. (1983). Reconsidering the Social Rejection of Ex–Mental Patients: Levels of Attitudinal Response. *American Journal of Community Psychology, 11*(3), 261–273.

Livingston, J., Rossiter, K., and Verdun-Jones, S. (2011). "Forensic" Labelling: An Empirical Assessment of its Effects on Self-Stigma for People with Severe Mental

Illness. *Psychiatry Research, 188*(1), 115–122.

Lomas, J. (2006). Commentary: Whose Views Count in Evidence Synthesis? And When Do They Count? *Healthcare Policy, 1*(2), 55–57.

Mancini, M., Hardiman, E., and Lawson, H. (2005). Making Sense of It All: Consumer Providers' Theories About Factors Facilitating and Impeding Recovery from Psychiatric Disabilities. *Psychiatric Rehabilitation Journal, 29*(1), 48–55.

Maslow, A. H. (1966). *The Psychology of Science: A Reconnaissance.* New York: Harper and Row.

Massey, J., Brooks, M., Burrow, J., and Sutherland, C. (2010). *Increasing Mental Health Literacy Among Student Affairs Staff: Assessing "Mental Health First Aid."* Kingston, Ontario: Queen's University.

McArthur, A., and Dunion, L. (2007). *A Fairer Future.* see me Scotland.

McLuhan, M. (1995). *The Essential McLuhan,* E. McLuhan, and F. Zingrone, eds. Toronto: Anansi Press.

Mechanic, D., and Rochefort, D. (1990). Deinstitutionalization: An Appraisal of Reform. *Annual Review of Sociology, 16,* 301–327.

Mental Health Commission of Canada. (2011, May 15). Retrieved from http://www. mentalhealthcommission.ca.

Ministry of Health of New Zealand. (2007). *Like Minds, Like Mine National Plan 2007– 2013: Programme to Counter Stigma and Discrimination Associated with Mental Illness.* Wellington, New Zealand: Ministry of Health.

Mohammad, A., Schur, L., and Blanck, P. (2011). What Types of Jobs Do People with Disabilities Want? *Journal of Occupational Rehabilitation, 21,* 199–210.

Morris, Z. S., and Clarkson, P. J. (2009). Does Social Marketing Provide a Framework for Changing Healthcare Practice? *Health Policy, 91,* 135–141.

Murdoch, J. (2000). Networks—A New Paradigm of Rural Development? *Journal of Rural Studies, 16,* 407–419.

Murray, C., and Lopez, A. (1996). *The Global Burden of Disease.* Geneva, Switzerland: World Health Orgnization.

Myers, F., Woodhouse, A., Whitehead, I., McCollam, A., McBryde, L., Pinfold, V., et al. (2009). *Evaluation of "See Me"—the National Scottish Campaign Against the Stigma and Discrimination Associated with Mental Ill-Health.* Edinburgh: Scottish Government Social Research.

Nasser, M. (1995). The Rise and Fall of Anti-Psychiatry. *Psychiatric Bulletin, 1995*(19), 743–746.

Ng, C. (1997). The Stigma of Mental Illness in Asian Cultures. *Australian and New Zealand Journal of Psychiatry, 31,* 382–390.

NIH. (2012, accessed January 29, 2012), http://222.nih.gov/about/director/ budgetrequest/HIH_BIB_020911.pdf

Nunes, J., and Simmie, S. (2002). *Beyond Crazy.* Toronto, Ontario: McClelland and Steward, Ltd.

Office of the Deputy Prime Minister. (2004). *Mental Health and Social Exclusion.* London: Office of the Deputy Prime Minister.

Okasha, A. (1999). Mental Health in the Middle East: An Egyptian Perspective. *Clinical Psychology Review, 19*(8), 917–933.

Okasha, A., Arboleda-Flórez, J., and Sartorius, N. (eds.). (2000). *Ethics, Culture and*

Psychiatry. Washington: APPI.

O'Keefe, E., and Hogg, C. (1999). Public Participation and Marginalized Groups: The Community Development Model. *Health Expectations, 2,* 245–254.

Paihez, G., Bulbena, A., Coll, J., Ros, S., and Balon, R. (2005). Attitudes and Views on Psychiatry: A Comparison Between Spanish and U.S. Medical Students. *Academic Psychiatry, 29,* 82–91.

Paluck, L, E., and Green, D. P. (2009). Prejudice Reduction: What Works? A Review and Assessment of Research and Practice. *Annual Review of Psychology, 60,* 339–367.

Pan, P., Lee, P., and Lei-Mak, F. (1990). Psychiatry as Compared to Other Career Choices: A Survey of Medical Students in Hong Kong. *Medical Education, 24,* 251–257.

Peattie, S., and Peattie, K. (2003). Ready to Fly Solo? Reducing Social Marketing's Dependence on Commercial Marketing Theory. *Marketing Theory, 3*(3), 365–385.

Pescosolido, B. A., Martin, J. K., Long, J. S., Medina, T. R., and Link, B. G. (2010). "A Disease Like Any Other"? A Decade of Change in Public Reactions to Schizophrenia, Depression, and Alcohol Dependence. *American Journal of Psychiatry in Advance* (September 15), 1–10.

Pescosolido, B., Monahan, J., Link, B., Stueve, A., and Kikuzawa, S. (1999). The Public's View of the Competence, Dangerousness, and Need for Legal Coercion of Persons with Mental Health Problems. *American Journal of Public Health, 89,* 1339–1345.

Phelan, J. (2005). Geneticization of Deviant Behaviour and Consequences for Stigma: The Case of Mental Illness. *Journal of Health and Social Behaviour, 46,* 307–322.

Phelan, J. C., Link, B. G., Stueve, A., and Pescosolido, B. A. (2000). Public Conceptions of Mental Illness in 1950 and 1996: What Is Mental Illness and Is It to Be Feared? *Journal of Health and Social Behavior, 41*(2), 188–207.

Phelan, J., Bromet, E., and Link, B. (1998). Psychiatric Illness and Family Stigma. *Schizophrenia Bulletin, 24*(1), 115–126.

Pinfold, V., Huxley, P., Thornicroft, G., Farmer, P., Toulmin, H., and Graham, T. (2003). Reducing Psychiatric Stigma and Discrimination: Evaluating an Educational Intervention with the Police Force in England. *Social Psychiatry and Psychiatric Epidemiology, 38,* 337–344.

Pirkis, J., Blood, R., Dare, A., and Holland, K. (2008). *The Media Monitoring Project: Changes in Media Reporting of Suicide and Mental Health and Illness in Australia: 2000/01–2006/07.* Canberra: Commonwealth of Australia.

Posavac, E. (2011). *Program Evaluation: Methods and Case Studies.* Upper Saddle River, NJ: Prentice Hall.

Powell, R., and Lloyd, K. R. (2001). A National Survey of Violence Experienced by Community Mental Health Researchers. *Social Psychiatry and Psychiatric Epidemiology, 36,* 158–163.

Psychiatric Times. (1991, accessed November 2, 2011). Prozac Frees Ex-Scientology Leader from Depression. *The Psychiatric Times,* http://www.mombu.com/ medicine/psychology/t-psychiatric-times-prozac-frees-ex-scientology-leader-from-depression-now-online-with-images-1907216.html

Raguram, R., Raghu, T., Vounatsou, P., and Weiss, M. (2004). Schizophrenia and the Cultural Epidemiology of Stigma in Bangalore, India. *Journal of Nervous and Mental Diseases, 192,* 734–744.

Raistrick, D., Russell, D., Tober, G., and Tindale, A. (2008). A Survey of Substance Use by Health Care Professionals and Their Attitudes to Substance Misuse Patients (NHS Staff Survey). *Journal of Substance Use, 13*(1), 57–69.

Rochefort, D. (1993). *From Poorhouses to Homelessness.* Westport, CT: Auburn House.

Rosenhan, D. (1974). On Being Sane in Insane Places. *Clinical Social Work Journal, 2,* 237–256.

Ross, C., and Goldner, E. (2009). Stigma, Negative Attitudes, and Discrimination Towards Mental Illness Within the Nursing Profession: A Review of the Literature. *Journal of Psychiatric and Mental Health Nursing, 16,* 558–567.

Rossi, P. H., Lipsey, M. W., and Freeman, H. E. (2004). *Evaluation: A Systematic Approach.* Thousand Oaks, California: Sage Publications.

SANE Australia. (2007). Retrieved February 1, 2007, from http:/www.sane.org.

Saraceno, B. (2005). The Role of Advocacy in Striving for a Significant Change: A WHO Partnership. In A. Okasha and C. Stefanis (eds.), *Perspectives on the Stigma of Mental Illness* (pp. 123–131). Geneva, Switzerland: World Psychiatric Association.

Sartorius, N. (1996). Long-Term Follow-up of Schizophrenia in 16 Countries: A Description of the International Study of Schizophrenia Conducted by the World Health Organization. *Social Psychiatry and Psychiatric Epidemiology, 31,* 249–258.

Sartorius, N. (1998). Stigma: What Can Psychiatrists Do About It? *The Lancet, 352,* 1058–1059.

Sartorius, N. (2002a). *Fighting for Mental Health: A Personal View.* Cambridge, England: Cambridge University Press.

Sartorius, N. (2002b). Iatrogenic Stigma of Mental Illness. *British Medical Journal, 324,* 1470–1471.

Sartorius, N. (2002c). The Mental Health Adventure of the World Health Organization. In N. Sartorius, *Fighting for Mental Health* (pp. 123–141). Cambridge, England: Cambridge University Press.

Sartorius, N. (2004). The World Psychiatric Association Programme Against Stigma and Discrimination Because of Schizophrenia. In A. Crisp (ed.), *Every Family in the Land* (pp. 373–375). London: Royal Society of Medicine Press.

Sartorius, N. (2006). Lessons from a 10-Year Global Program Against Stigma and Discriminiation Because of an Illness. *Psychology, Health and Medicine, 11*(3), 383–388.

Sartorius, N. (2010). Short-Lived Campaigns Are Not Enough. *Nature, 468,* 163–165.

Sartorius, N., and Schulze, H. (2005). *Reducing the Stigma of Mental Illness.* Cambridge, England: Cambridge University Press.

Sartorius, N., Gaebel, W., Cleveland, H., Stuart, H., Akiyama, T., Arboleda-Flórez, J., et al. (2010). WPA Guidance on How to Combat Stigmatization of Psychiatry and Psychiatrists. *World Psychiatry, 9,* 131–144.

Sayce, L., and Curran, C. (2005). Tackling Social Exclusion Across Europe. In M. Knapp, D. McDaid, E. Mossialos, and G. Thornicroft (eds.), *Mental Health Policy and Practice Across Europe* (pp. 34–59). Berkshire, England: McGraw-Hill Open University Press.

Scheff, T. (1966). *Being Mentally Ill: A Sociological Theory.* Chicago, IL: Aldine.

Schoen, C., Osborn, R., Huynh, P., Doty, M., Peugh, J., and Zapert, K. (2006). On the Front Lines of Care: Primary Care Doctors' Office Systems, Experiences, and Views in Seven Countries. *Health Affairs, 25,* w555–w571.

Schulze, B. (2007). Stigma and Mental Health Professionals. A Review of the Evidence on an Intricate Relationship. *International Review of Psychiatry, 19*, 137–155.

Schulze, B., and Angermeyer, M. C. (2003). Subjective Experiences of Stigma. A Focus Group Study of Schizophrenic Patients, Their Relatives and Mental Health Professionals. *Social Science and Medicine, 56*, 299–312.

Schur, L., Kruse, D., Blasi, J., and Blanck, P. (2009). Is Disability Disabling in All Workplaces? Workplace Disparities and Corporate Culture. *Industrial Relations, 48*(3), 381–410.

Schütz, H., and Six, B. (1996). How Strong Is the Relationship Between Prejudice and Discrimination? A Meta-Analytic Answer. *International Journal of Intercultural Relations, 20*, 441–462.

Scriven, M. (1991). *Evaluation Thesaurus* (4th Ed.). Newbury Park, CA: Sage Publications.

Sealy, P., and Whitehead, P. (2004). Forty Years of Deinstitutionalization of Psychiatric Services in Canada: An Empirical Assessment. *Canadian Journal of Psychiatry, 49*(4), 249–257.

Sharfstein, S., and Dickerson, F. (2006). Psychiatry and the Consumer Movement. *Health Affairs, 25*(3), 734–736.

Shorter, E. (2007). The Historical Development of Mental Health Services in Europe. In M. Knapp, D. McDaid, E. Mossialos, and G. Thornicroft (eds.), *Mental Health Policy and Practice Across Europe* (pp. 15–33). Berkshire, England: McGraw-Hill Open Unviersity Press.

Shortt, S. (1986). *Victorian Lunacy.* Cambridge, England: Cambridge University Press.

Shortt, S., Hwang, S., Stuart, H., Bedore, M., Zurba, N., and Darling, M. (2008). Delivering Primary Care to Homeless Persons: A Policy Analysis Approach to Evaluating the Options. *Healthcare Policy, 4*(1), 108–122.

Simmie, S., and Nunes, J. (2001). *The Last Taboo: A Survival Guide to Mental Health Care in Canada.* Toronto, Ontario: McClelland and Stewart, Ltd.

Simon, B. (1992). Shame, Stigma, and Mental Illness in Ancient Greece. In P. Fink and A. Tasman (eds.), *Stigma and Mental Illness.* Washington, DC: American Psychiatric Press.

Standing Committee on Social Affairs, Science and Technology. (2006). *Out of the Shadows at Last: Transforming Mental Health, Mental Illness, and Addictions Services in Canada.* Ottawa: The Parliament of Canada.

Stead, M., Hastings, G., and McDermott, L. (2007). The Meaning, Effectiveness and Future of Social Marketing. *Obesity Reviews, 8*(Suppl. 1), 189–193.

Steadman, H. (1972). The Psychiatrist as a Conservative Agent of Social Control. *Social Problems, 20*(2), 263–271.

Stefanis, C., and Economou, M. (2005). The Unprecedented Initiative of European Ministers of Health. In A. Okasha and C. Stefanis (eds.), *Perspectives on the Stigma of Mental Illness* (pp. 7–20). Geneva, Switzerland: World Psychiatric Association.

Stewart, W., Ricci, J., Chee, E., Hahn, S., and Morganstein, D. (2003). Cost of Lost Productive Work Time Among U.S. Workers with Depression. *JAMA, 289*, 3135–3144.

Streiner, D., and Norman, G. (1995). *Health Measurement Scales: A Practical Guide to Their Development and Use* (2nd Ed.). Oxford, England: Oxford University Press.

Stuart, H. (2003a). Stigma and the Daily News: Evaluation of a Newspaper Intervention. *Canadian Journal of Psychiatry, 48*, 651–656.

Stuart, H. (2003b). Violence and Mental Illness: An Overview. *World Psychiatry, 2*(2), 121–124.

Stuart, H. (2006a). Media Portrayal of Mental Illness and Its Treatments: What Effect Does It Have on People with Mental Illness? *CNS Drugs, 20*(2), 99–106.

Stuart, H. (2006b). Mental Illness and Employment Discrimination. *Current Opinion in Psychiatry, 19*, 522–526.

Stuart, H. (2006c). Reaching Out to High School Youth: The Effectiveness of a Video-Based Anti-Stigma Program. *Canadian Journal of Psychiatry, 51*, 647–653.

Stuart, H. (2007). Employment Equity and Mental Disability. *Current Opinion in Psychiatry, 20*, 486–490.

Stuart, H. (2008). Building an Evidence Base for Anti-Stigma Programming. In J. Arboleda-Flórez and N. Sartorius (eds.), *Understanding the Stigma of Mental Illness: Theory and Interventions* (pp. 135–145). London: John Wiley and Sons, Ltd.

Stuart, H. (2009). Stigma and Discrimination. In G. Christodoulou, M. Jorge, and J. Mezzich (eds.), *Advances in Psychiatry, Volume 3* (pp. 211–217). Athens, Greece: Beta Medical Publishers.

Stuart, H. (2010). Canadian Perspectives on Stigma Because of Mental Illness. In D. Streiner and J. Cairney (eds.), *Mental Disorders in Canada: An Epidemiologic Perspective.* (pp. 304–330) Toronto, Ontario: University of Toronto Press.

Stuart, H., and Arboleda-Flórez, J. (2000). Homeless Shelter Users in the Post-Deinstitutionalization Era. *Canadian Journal of Psychiatry, 45*, 55–62.

Stuart, H., and Arboleda-Flórez, J. (2001). Community Attitudes Toward People with Schizophrenia. *Canadian Journal of Psychiatry, 46*, 245–252.

Stuart, H., Koller, M., Christie, R., and Pietrus, M. (2011). Reducing Mental Health Stigma: A Case Study. *Healthcare Quarterly, 14*(Special Issue [April]), 41–49.

Stuart, H., Milev, R., and Koller, M. (2005). The Inventory of Stigmatizing Experiences: Its Development and Reliability. *World Psychiatry, 4*(S1), 35–39.

Swartz, M., Swanson, J., and Hannon, M. (2003). Does Fear of Coercion Keep People Away from Mental Health Treatment? Evidence from a Survey of Persons with Schizophrenia and Mental Health Professionals. *Behavioral Sciences and the Law, 21*, 459–472.

Szasz, T. (1960). The Myth of Mental Illness. *American Psychologist, 15*, 113–118.

Szasz, T. (1974). *The Myth of Mental Illness: Foundations of a Theory of Personal Conduct* (Revised Ed.). New York: Harper and Row.

Szasz, T. (1977). *Psychiatric Slavery: When Confinement and Coercion Masquerade as Cure.* New York: Free Press.

Szasz, T. (2007). *Coercion as Cure: A Critical History of Psychiatry.* New Brunswick, NJ: Transaction Publishers.

Tagliaventi, M., and Mattarelli, E. (2006). The Role of Networks of Practice, Value Sharing, and Operational Proximity in Knowledge Flows Between Professional Groups. *Human Relations, 59*(3), 291–319.

Takahashi, L. (1997). Information and Attitudes Toward Mental Health Care Facilities: Implications for Addressing the NIMBY Syndrome. *Journal of Planning Education and Research, 17*, 119–130.

BIBLIOGRAPHY AND SUGGESTED READINGS

Thara, R., and Srinivasan, T.N. (2000). How Stigmatizing Is Schizophrenia in India? *International Journal of Social Psychiatry, 46*(2), 135–141.

Thornicroft, G. (2006). *Shunned. Discrimination Against People with Mental Illness.* Oxford, England: Oxford University Press.

Thornicroft, G., Brohan, E., Rose, D., Sartorius, N., Leese, M., and INDIGO Study Group. (2009). Global Pattern of Experienced and Anticipated Discrimination Against People with Schizophrenia: A Cross-Sectional Survey. *Lancet, 373*, 408–415.

Thornicroft, G., Rose, D., and Kassam, A. (2007). Discrimination in Health Care Against People with Mental Illness. *International Review of Psychiatry, 19*(2), 113–122.

Thornicroft, G., Rose, D., and Mehta, N. (2010). Discrimination Against People with Mental Illness: What Can Psychiatrists Do? *Advances in Psychiatric Treatment, 16*, 53–59.

Tolomiczenko, G., Goering, P., and Durbin, J. (2001). Educating the Public About Mental Illness and Homelessness: A Cautionary Note. *Canadian Journal of Psychiatry, 46*, 253–257.

Tomes, H. (2006). The Patient as a Policy Factor: A Historical Case Study of the Consumer/Survivor Movement in Mental Health. *Health Affairs, 25*(3), 720–729.

Torrey, E. (2010). Patients, Clients, Consumers, Survivors, et al: What's In a Name? *Schizophrenia Bulletin, 37*(3), 466–468.

Torrey, F. (1995). *Surviving Schizophrenia: A Manual for Families, Consumers and Providers* (5th Ed.). New York: Harper and Row.

Tsang, H., Angell, B., Corrigan, P., Lee, Y., Shi, K., Lam, C., et al. (2007). A Cross-Cultural Study of Employers' Concerns About Hiring People with a Psychotic Disorder: Implications for Recovery. *Social Psychiatry and Psychiatric Epidemiology, 42*, 723–733.

Tzeng, W., and Lipson, J. (2004). The Cultural Context of Suicide Stigma in Taiwan. *Qualitative Health Research, 14*(3), 345–358.

United Nations General Assembly. (1991). A/RES/46/119 Geneva: United Nations

United Nations General Assembly. (2006, December 13). *Convention on the Rights of Persons with Disabilities (CRPD).* Geneva: United Nations.

Ustun, B., and Sartorius, N. (eds.). (1995). *Mental Illness in General Health Care.* Chichester, England: John Wiley and Sons.

Wahl, O. (1999). *Telling Is Risky Business.* New Brunswick, NJ: Rutgers University Press.

Weatherhead, S., and Daiches, A. (2010). Muslim View on Mental Health and Psychotherapy. *Psychology and Psychotherapy: Theory, Research and Practice, 83*, 75–89.

Wedding, D., Boyd, M., and Niemec Niemiec, R. (2005). *Movies and Mental Illness* (2nd Revised Ed.). Cambridge, MA: Hogrefe and Huber, Publishers.

Wegerif, R. (1998). The Social Dimension of Asynchronous Learning Networks. *Journal of Asynchronous Learning Networks, 2*, 34–49.

Weiss, C. (1995). Nothing as Practical as Good Theory: Exploring Theory-based Evaluation for Comprehensive Community Initiatives for Children and Families. In J. Connell, A. Kubisch, L. Schorr, and C. Weiss (eds.), *New Approaches to Evaluating Community Initiatives* (pp. 65–92). Washington, DC: The Aspen Institute.

Weiss, M., Sharma, S., Gaur, R., Sahrma, J., Desai, A., and Doongaji, D. (1986). Traditional Concepts of Mental Disorder Among Indian Psychiatric Patients: Prelimnary Report of a Work in Progress. *Social Science and Medicine, 23*(4), 379–386.

WHO Mental Health Survey Consortium. (2005). Prevalence, Severity, and Unmet Need for Treatment of Mental Disorders in the World Health Organization World Mental Health Surveys. *JAMA 291*(21), 2581–2590.

Wolf, G., Pathare, S., Craig, T., and Leff, J. (1999). Public Education for Community Care: A New Approach. In J. Guimon, W. Fischer, and N. Sartorius (eds.), *The Image of Madness* (pp. 105–117). Basil, Switzerland: Karger.

World Health Organization. (2001). *Mental Health: A Call for Action by World Health Ministers.* Geneva, Switzerland: World Health Organization.

World Health Organization. (2001). *Results of a Global Advocacy Campaign.* Geneva: World Health Organization.

World Health Organization. (2001). *The World Health Report 2001. Mental Health: New Understanding, New Hope.* Geneva: World Health Organization.

World Health Organization. (2003). *Investing in Mental Health.* Geneva: World Health Organization.

World Health Organization. (2005). *Mental Health Atlas 2005* (Revised Ed.). Geneva: World Health Organization.

World Health Organization and the World Bank. (2011). *World Report on Disability.* Geneva: World Health Organization.

World Psychiatric Association Global Program to Reduce Stigma and Discrimination Because of Schizophrenia. (2005). *Schizophrenia—Open the Doors Training Manual.* Geneva: Open the Doors, World Psychiatric Association.

Wyllie, A., and Mackinlay, C. (2007). *Impacts of National Media Campaign to Counter Stigma and Discrimination Associated with Mental Illness.* Wellington: New Zealand Ministry of Health.

APPENDIX

Inventories of Stigma Experiences

These semi-structured interviews can be used, with permission of the authors, to elicit stigmatizing experiences from people who have a mental illness and their family members. Information obtained can be used to guide anti-stigma program interventions. The interviews also contain two scales to measure the frequency and psychosocial impact of stigma. They are available in several languages. Information on the psychometric qualities of the frequency and impact scales and their scoring can be found in H. Stuart, M. Koller, and R. Milev (2008), "Inventories to Measure the Scope and Impact of Stigma Experiences from the Perspective of Those Who Are Stigmatized—Consumer and Family," in, J. Arboleda-Flórez and N. Sartorius (eds.), *Understanding the Stigma of Mental Illness: Theory and Interventions* (pp. 193–204), West Sussex, England: John Wiley & Sons, Ltd.

PERSONAL EXPERIENCES WITH THE
STIGMA OF MENTAL ILLNESS[1]

> **Information about you**
>
> First, we would like to know a bit about you and your contact with mental
> health treatment services. Please mark the correct box.

1. **Gender**   □ Male   □ Female

2. **What year were you born?** _____

3. **What is your highest level of education?**

   □ Public school or less (up to grade 8)
   □ Some high school
   □ Completed high school (grade 12 or 13)
   □ Some college or technical training
   □ Completed college or technical training
   □ Some university
   □ Completed university
   □ Graduate or professional degree

4. **Are you currently living alone or with someone else?**

   □ Alone
   □ Spouse/partner
   □ Parents
   □ Other relative(s)
   □ Other unrelated person(s)
   □ Other Specify _____

5. **What is your current marital status?**

   □ Never married
   □ Separated
   □ Widowed
   □ Divorced
   □ Common/law
   □ Married

---

[1] © H. Stuart (heather.stuart@queensu.ca), R. Milev, M. Koller Suggested Citation: Stuart H,
Milev R, Koller M. (2005) The Inventory of Stigma Experiences: Development and Reliability.
World Psychiatry, Vol. 4(Supplement 1): 33–37. To be used with the permission of the authors.

6. **Are you employed?**
    - ☐ Not employed
        - ○ Unable to work because of mental health problems
        - ○ Unable to work because of other health problems
        - ○ Homemaker
        - ○ Retired
        - ○ Student
        - ○ Volunteer
    - ☐ Supported employment
    - ☐ Part-time competitive work
    - ☐ Full-time competitive work

Information about your mental health problems.

This section asks about your mental health problems and the kinds of services you may have used.

---

7. **What is your current diagnosis (check more than one if applicable)?**
    - ☐ None
    - ☐ Schizophrenia
    - ☐ Manic Depression/Bipolar Disorder
    - ☐ Depression
    - ☐ Anxiety Disorder
    - ☐ Misuse of alcohol or street drugs
    - ☐ Other: Specify _____

8. **Compared to one year ago, would you say your mental illness is . . .**
    - ☐ Better
    - ☐ About the same
    - ☐ Worse

9. **How old were you when you first noticed you had symptoms?**

    _____

10. **How old were you when you first received treatment?**

    _____

11. **Would you say that you have come to accept your diagnosis?**
    - ☐ No
    - ☐ Yes, If yes, how old were you when accepted your diagnosis?

12. **Have you ever been hospitalized for a mental illness or suicide attempt?**

☐ Yes
☐ No

12a) Have you ever been hospitalized in:

☐ A provincial psychiatric hospital
☐ A general hospital psychiatric unit
☐ A medical/surgical unit in a general hospital

12b) Were you ever committed under Provincial mental health legislation (the Mental Health Act)?

☐ Yes
☐ No
☐ Uncertain

12c) Have you been hospitalized in the last year because of a mental health problem?

☐ Yes, as a voluntary patient
☐ Yes, as a committed patient
☐ No

12d) Have you ever been hospitalized on a forensic unit?

☐ Yes
☐ No
☐ Uncertain

13. **In the last year have you attended an outpatient or community mental health program?**

☐ No
☐ Yes. About how often do you attend?
  ○ Weekly or more often
  ○ 2 or 3 times a month
  ○ Once a month
  ○ Once every 2 or 3 months
  ○ Once every 6 months
  ○ Once or twice a year

Experiences with Stigma

The next section asks about your experiences with stigma. By stigma we mean negative feelings people have toward people with a mental or emotional disorder.

The next questions will ask about your own personal experiences with stigma.

14. **Do you think that people will think less of you if they know you have a mental or emotional disorder?**

    □ Never
    □ Rarely
    □ Sometimes
    □ Often
    □ Always

15. **Do you think that the average person is afraid of someone with a serious mental illness?**

    □ Never
    □ Rarely
    □ Sometimes
    □ Often
    □ Always

16. **Have you ever been teased, bullied, or harassed because you have a mental or emotional disorder?**

    □ No
    □ Unsure
    □ Yes

    Please explain.

    _____
    _____
    _____
    _____
    _____

17.   **Have you felt that you have been treated unfairly or that your rights have been denied because you have a mental or emotional disorder?**

    □ No
    □ Unsure
    □ Yes

Please explain.

_____

_____

_____

_____

_____

18.   **Could you give us an example of a stigmatizing experience you have had in the last year?**

_____

_____

_____

_____

_____

_____

_____

19.   **Was this the worst experience of stigma you have ever had?**

    □ Yes
    □ No. If not, what was the worst stigmatizing experience you have ever had?

_____

_____

_____

_____

_____

20.   **When did this happen?** _____

21. **Have your experiences with stigma affected your recovery?**

   ☐ No
   ☐ Not sure
   ☐ Yes. If yes, could you give us an example?

   _____
   _____
   _____
   _____
   _____
   _____

22. **Have your experiences with stigma caused you to think less about yourself or your abilities?**

   ☐ No
   ☐ Unsure
   ☐ Yes

   If yes, could you give us an example of how you have been affected?

   _____
   _____
   _____
   _____
   _____

23. **Have your experiences with stigma affected your ability to make or keep friends?**

   ☐ No
   ☐ Unsure
   ☐ Yes

   Could you explain?

   _____
   _____
   _____
   _____

24. **Have your experiences with stigma affected your ability to interact with your family?**

     ☐ No
     ☐ Unsure
     ☐ Yes

Could you explain?

_____

_____

_____

_____

_____

25. **Have your experiences with stigma affected your satisfaction with or quality of life?**

     ☐ No
     ☐ Unsure
     ☐ Yes

Could you explain?

_____

_____

_____

_____

_____

26. **Do you think your family been stigmatized because of your mental illness?**

     ☐ N/A – No family contact
     ☐ No
     ☐ Unsure
     ☐ Yes

If yes, could you give us an example of how your family has been affected?

_____

_____

_____

_____

_____

27.   **What do you do to cope with stigma?**

_____

_____

_____

_____

_____

_____

28.   **Do you try to conceal your mental or emotional disorder from others?**

☐ No
☐ Unsure
☐ Yes

Could you explain?

_____

_____

_____

_____

_____

_____

29.   **Do you try to avoid situations that may be stigmatizing to you?**

☐ No
☐ Unsure
☐ Yes

Could you explain?

_____

_____

_____

_____

_____

_____

30.   **Have you ever tried to reduce stigma by educating your friends or family about your mental or emotional disorder?**

☐ No
☐ Unsure
☐ Yes

Could you explain?

_____

_____

_____

_____

_____

31.   **Have your experiences with stigma motivated you to speak out about the rights of the mentally ill?**

☐ No
☐ Unsure
☐ Yes

Could you explain?

_____

_____

_____

_____

_____

32.   **Have your experiences with stigma motivated you to participate in programs to educate the public about mental illness.**

☐ No
☐ Unsure
☐ Yes

Could you explain?

_____

_____

_____

_____

_____

33.   **On a ten-point scale where 0 is the lowest possible amount, and 10 is the highest possible amount, how much has stigma negatively affected you personally? Please circle the number that best quantifies this impact in the following areas.**

Quality of Life: _____

              0   1   2   3   4   5   6   7   8   9   10

Social Contacts: _____

              0   1   2   3   4   5   6   7   8   9   10

Family Relations: _____

              0   1   2   3   4   5   6   7   8   9   10

Self Esteem: _____

              0   1   2   3   4   5   6   7   8   9   10

34.   **On a ten-point scale where 0 is the lowest possible amount, and 10 is the highest possible amount, how much has stigma negatively affected your family as a whole? Please circle the number that best quantifies this impact in the following areas. If you do not have contact with your family, circle N/A. If you don't know, circle DK.**

Quality of Life: _____

N/A   DK   0   1   2   3   4   5   6   7   8   9   10

Social Contacts: _____

N/A   DK   0   1   2   3   4   5   6   7   8   9   10

Family Relations: _____

N/A   DK   0   1   2   3   4   5   6   7   8   9   10

35. **What do you think causes stigma?**

_____

_____

_____

_____

_____

_____

_____

36. **What should we do to fight stigma?**

_____

_____

_____

_____

_____

_____

_____

Thank you for taking your time to talk with us. Is there anything else you would like us to know about your experiences with stigma that we have not yet asked?

Additional Comments:

_____

_____

_____

_____

_____

_____

_____

_____

FAMILY EXPERIENCES WITH THE STIGMA
OF MENTAL ILLNESS[2]

Information about you

First, we would like to know a bit about you. Please mark the correct box.

---

1. **Gender**   ☐ Male   ☐ Female

2. **What year were you born?** _____

3. **What is your highest level of education?**

    ☐ Public school or less (up to grade 8)
    ☐ Some high school
    ☐ Completed high school (grade 12 or 13)
    ☐ Some college or technical training
    ☐ Completed college or technical training
    ☐ Some university
    ☐ Completed university
    ☐ Graduate or professional degree

4. **What is your current living arrangement? Are you currently living . . .**

    ☐ Alone
    ☐ With a Spouse/partner
    ☐ With Parents
    ☐ With another relative(s)
    ☐ With other unrelated person(s)
    ☐ Other Specify _____

5. **Are you employed?**

    ☐ Not employed
    ☐ Homemaker
    ☐ Retired
    ☐ Student
    ☐ Volunteer
    ☐ Employed Full-time
    ☐ Employed Part-time

---

[2] © H. Stuart (heather.stuart@queensu.ca), R. Milev, M. Koller Suggested Citation: Stuart H, Milev R, Koller M. (2005) The Inventory of Stigma Experiences: Development and Reliability. *World Psychiatry*, Vol. 4(Supplement 1): 33–37. To be used with the permission of the authors.

Information about your relative's mental health problems.

6. **Does your relative currently have any of the following illnesses? (check as many as apply).**

    ☐ Schizophrenia
    ☐ Manic Depression/Bipolar Disorder
    ☐ Depression
    ☐ Anxiety Disorder
    ☐ Misuse of alcohol or street drugs
    ☐ Other: Specify _____

7. **What is your relationship to this person?**

    Relationship: _____

8. **Does your relative currently live with you?**

    ☐ Yes
    ☐ Yes, but currently in hospital
    ☐ No

9. **How old is your relative?**

    Age at last birthday: _____

10. **Are they ...**

    ☐ Male
    ☐ Female

11. **Compared to <u>one year ago</u>, would you say their mental illness is ...**

    ☐ Better
    ☐ About the same
    ☐ Worse

12. **About how old were they when they first had symptoms?**

    _____

13. **About how old were they when they first received treatment?**

    _____

14. **Have they ever been hospitalized for a mental illness or suicide attempt?**

☐ Yes
☐ No
☐ Don't know

14a) Have they ever been hospitalized in:

☐ A provincial psychiatric hospital
☐ A general hospital psychiatric unit
☐ A medical/surgical unit in a general hospital
☐ Don't know

14b) Have they ever been involuntarily admitted under mental health legislation (eg: a Mental Health Act)?

☐ Yes
☐ No
☐ Uncertain

14c) Have they been hospitalized in the last year because of a mental health problem?

☐ Yes, as a voluntary patient
☐ Yes, as a committed patient
☐ No
☐ Don't know

14d) Have you ever been personally involved in a family member's involuntary admission process?

☐ Yes
☐ No
☐ Uncertain

14e) Have they ever been hospitalized in a forensic unit for people who have a mental illness and are involved with the law?

☐ Yes
☐ No
☐ Uncertain

15. **In the last year have they attended an outpatient or community mental health program?**

    ☐ Don't know

    ☐ No

    ☐ Yes.

        If yes, about how often do they attend?

           ○ Weekly or more often

           ○ 2 or 3 times a month

           ○ Once a month

           ○ Once every 2 or 3 months

           ○ Once every 6 months

           ○ Once or twice a year

Experiences with Stigma

The next section asks about experiences with stigma you or your family as a whole has had.

By stigma we mean negative feelings people have toward people with a mental illness that may result in unfair treatment or discrimination.

---

16. **Do you think that people think less of those who have a mental illness?**

    ☐ Never

    ☐ Rarely

    ☐ Sometimes

    ☐ Often

    ☐ Always

17. **Do you think that the average person is afraid of someone with a serious mental illness?**

    ☐ Never

    ☐ Rarely

    ☐ Sometimes

    ☐ Often

    ☐ Always

18. **Has your relative been stigmatized because of their mental illness?**

   ☐ Never
   ☐ Rarely
   ☐ Sometimes
   ☐ Often
   ☐ Always

   Please explain.

   _____

   _____

   _____

   _____

19. **Have you felt stigmatized because of your relative's mental illness?**

   ☐ Never
   ☐ Rarely
   ☐ Sometimes
   ☐ Often
   ☐ Always

   Please explain.

   _____

   _____

   _____

   _____

20. **Have other members of your family been stigmatized because of your relative's mental illness?**

   ☐ Never
   ☐ Rarely
   ☐ Sometimes
   ☐ Often
   ☐ Always

   Please explain.

   _____

   _____

   _____

   _____

21. **Could you give us an example of a stigmatizing experience your family has had in the last year?**

_____
_____
_____
_____
_____
_____

22. **Was this the worst experience of stigma your family has had?**

□ Yes

□ No. If not, what was the worst stigmatizing experience you or your family has had?

_____
_____
_____
_____
_____
_____

23. **When did this happen?** _____

24. **What impact has stigma had on your family?**

_____
_____
_____
_____
_____

25. **Have stigma affected your family's ability to make or keep friends?**

    ☐ Yes
    ☐ No
    ☐ Not sure

    Could you explain?

    _____
    _____
    _____
    _____
    _____

26. **Has stigma affected your ability to interact with your other relatives?**

    ☐ Yes
    ☐ No
    ☐ Not sure

    Could you explain?

    _____
    _____
    _____
    _____
    _____

27. **Have your experiences with stigma affected your family's quality of life?**

    ☐ Yes
    ☐ No
    ☐ Not sure

    Could you explain?

    _____
    _____
    _____
    _____
    _____

28.   **What does your family do to cope with stigma?**

_____

_____

_____

_____

_____

29.   **Do you try to avoid situations that may be stigmatizing to your family?**

□ Yes

□ No

□ Not sure

Could you explain?

_____

_____

_____

_____

_____

30.   **Have you ever tried to reduce stigma by educating your friends or relatives about mental illness?**

□ Yes

□ No

□ Not sure

Could you explain?

_____

_____

_____

_____

_____

31. **Have your experiences with stigma motivated a member of your family to speak out about the rights of the mentally ill?**

    ☐ Yes
    ☐ No
    ☐ Not sure

Could you explain?

_____

_____

_____

_____

32. **Have your experiences with stigma motivated a member of your family to participate in programs to educate the public about mental illness.**

    ☐ Yes
    ☐ No
    ☐ Not sure

Could you explain?

_____

_____

_____

_____

33. **On a ten-point scale where 0 is the lowest possible amount, and 10 is the highest possible amount, how much has stigma affected you personally? Please circle the number that best quantifies this impact in the following areas.**

Quality of Life: _____

    0 1 2 3 4 5 6 7 8 9 10

Social Contacts: _____

    0 1 2 3 4 5 6 7 8 9 10

Family Relations: _____

    0 1 2 3 4 5 6 7 8 9 10

Self Esteem: _____

    0 1 2 3 4 5 6 7 8 9 10

34. **On a ten-point scale where 0 is the lowest possible amount, and 10 is the highest possible amount, how much has stigma negatively affected your family as a whole? Please circle the number that best quantifies this impact in the following areas. Please circle N/A if you do not have contact with your family member who has a mental illness and DK if you don't know.**

Quality of Life: _____

N/A   DK   0   1   2   3   4   5   6   7   8   9   10

Social Contacts: _____

N/A   DK   0   1   2   3   4   5   6   7   8   9   10

Family Relations: _____

N/A   DK   0   1   2   3   4   5   6   7   8   9   10

35. **What do you think causes stigma?**

_____

_____

_____

_____

36. **What should we do to fight stigma?**

_____

_____

_____

_____

Thank you for taking your time to complete this survey. Is there anything else you would like us to know about your experiences with stigma that we have not yet asked?

Additional Comments:

_____

_____

_____

_____

_____

INDEX

Note: Page numbers followed by "*f*" and "*t*" refer to figures and tables, respectively.

abnormality, 76–77
abuse, 32, 87
active rehabilitation, 95
administrative governance, 45
advertising, 18, 166
advisory committee, 137–38
advocacy groups, 57
Africa, 12*f*
Allah, 34
All in the Family, 71
Amok, 37
anonymity, 178–79
anti-discrimination programs, 10
anti-psychiatry movement, 5–6,
    15, 105–8
anti-stigma programs, 8–9, 10, 16–19, 63.
    See also evaluation; semi-structured
    interviews
  activities that change behavior in, 48,
    127–28
  advisory committee of, 137–38
  building better practices for, 49, 53–56
  choosing an approach for, 160–63
  communicating results of, 180
  creating interest in, 139–40
  defining success of, 81–84
  documentation in, 49
  duration of, 129*t*
  endpoint of, 73
  enlightened opportunism and, 41–44, 49,
    68, 127
  family and, 164–65
  finances, 140–43
  focus groups, 145–47, 148*f*–149*f*, 150
  funding application for, 141–42
  goals of, 48–49, 129*t*, 130*t*, 138–39*f*, 162–63
  institutional racism in, 84–85
  knowledge-attitude-behavior continuum
    in, 78–79*f*
  leadership in, 45–47, 127
  legal provisions of, 130*t*, 132
  literature, 83, 161
  media usage in, 165–66
  medical knowledge and, 76–77
  mental health professionals and,
    57–59
  mental illness experience and delivery of,
    163–64
  monitoring of, 51–52, 140–43, 169–70
  neighborhood, 113–14, 159
  outcomes, 172–74
  paradigms and components of, 129*t*–130*t*,
    131–32
  people first in, 47
  perception of scientific evidence in, 51–52
  performance standards of, 82
  pilot-testing, 167*f*, 176
  planners, 70–71
  prejudice and, 67–69
  principles of, 47–49
  program committee for, 135, 136*f*, 137
  program logic model of, 161, 162*f*, 163
  qualitative investigation and priorities of,
    144–50
  resource acquisition and monitoring,
    140–43
  scientific evidence-based advocacy for,
    50–51, 55
  scope of, 129*t*, 131
  short-term, 96
  social-marketing campaign benchmarks
    for, 100*t*
  social-marketing campaign for, 70–71
  solutions, 70–71

anti-stigma programs (*Cont.*)
  sustainability of, 47–48
  target groups, 156–60
  targeting, 48, 127–28, 129*t*, 131
  targeting local needs in, 52–53, 126
  targeting media, 120–22
  task-oriented, 137
  universal, 92, 96–97, 102
  working with existing, 141
anxiety, 71
arbitrary detention, 20
arts, 166
asylums, 4. *See also* hospitals
  cage beds, 104, 105*f*
  in Canada, 87
  conditions of, 104
  early, 91
  European, 33
  forced confinement and treatment, 103–4,
    105*f*, 111
  Friern Hospital, 86
  Indian, 39
  Islamic, 33
  purpose of, 61
  Tooting Bec Hospital, 113–14
*Asylums: Essays on the Social Situation of
    Mental Patients and Other Inmates*
    (Goffman), 5, 88
attitude, 78, 85, 127–28
  assessing change in, 81–84
  etiological theories and, 110
  knowledge-attitude-behavior continuum,
    78–79*f*
  of mental health professionals, 63–64
  toward mental illness, Canadian, 88
  prejudice reduction, 79–81
attribution theory, 6–7
Australia, 37
  deinstitutionalization in, 89
  treatment in, 93
autonomy, 94

Balinese culture, stigma in, 38
A Beautiful Mind, 121
behavior, 76
  anti-stigma programs to change, 48, 127–28
  changing, 99, 101
  evaluation of, 173*f*
  knowledge-attitude-behavior continuum,
    78–79*f*

mental illness and, 69–70
  normality and, 68–69
Beyondblue: The National Depression Initiative,
    73–74
black box evaluation, 170
Blackfoot, 67–70, 76
black magic, 38
brainwashing, 29

cage bed, 104, 105*f*
Canada, 116–17, 121
  asylums in, 87
  deinstitutionalization in, 89
Canadian Alliance on Mental Illness and
    Mental Health, 71
Canadian Legion, 68
Canadian Medical Association, 71
Canadian Medical Association Journal, 15
Canadian Pilot Project, 115
cancer, 5
Carter Center, 121
checklist, focus group, 149*f*
China
  health-care systems in, 31
  knowledge of mental illness in, 37*t*
  recovery philosophy in, 37*t*
  social distance in, 36, 37*t*, 38
  stigma in culture of, 35–36, 37*t*, 38
Chinese medicine, 35
Church of Scientology, 107–8
civil commitment, 61–62, 108
civil rights. *See* rights
*Closed Ranks: An Experiment in Mental Health
    Education* (Cumming & Cumming), 68
  Blackfoot, 67–70, 76
CNN effect, 99
coercive treatment, 58, 62–63, 103–4, 105*f*, 128
  human rights and, 107
  survivors of, 106
cognitive-therapy intervention, 74
collaboration, 44
collectivist, 34
commercial marketing, 99–102, 100*t*
community-based programs, 41–42, 44, 57,
    63, 159
community care
  stigma and, 87*f*, 91–94
  transinstitutionalization and, 91–92
  treatment, 92–93
community development, 43, 46, 122

Community Health Centers Act (1963), 89
community-level interventions, 42–43
Community Mental Health Centers, 87
community projects, 122–24
community psychiatry, 91
community service development, 24
community treatment orders, 104
comparison groups, 179
concealment, of mental illness, 11
confidentiality, 178–79
confinement, 103–4, 105f, 111
Confucianism, 35
consent form, focus group, 148f
consumer-survivor groups, 107
Council of European Ministers, 112
courtesy stigma, 11, 11n2
    wise normals, 11n2
criminality, 28
cultures
    arts, 166
    social-marketing campaign and, 102
    society and, 102
    stigma in Balinese, 38
    stigma in Chinese, 35–36, 37t, 38
    stigma in Indian, 38–40
    stigma in Islamic, 33–35
    stigma in other, 33–40, 125–26
Cumming, E., 68–69
Cumming, J., 68–69

dangerousness, 61–62, 66, 72, 128
    public perceptions of, 108, 109f
    stereotype of, 100
de facto leaders, 46
degeneracy theory, 4
deinstitutionalization, 27, 128
    consequences of, 95
    target for, 89
demystification, 71
depression, 4, 12, 22, 24, 60, 71
    long-term outcomes of, 59
    recognition of, 73–74
    recovery from, 59
    treatment of, 73
developing countries, 31–33
development leaders, 46
diagnosis. See also labeling
    careless use of, 64
    effectiveness of, 88
    identity and, 58, 64

diagnostic overshadowing, 60, 93
disabilities
    civil rights and, 30
    employment and, 22–24
    mental illness and, 12–13
disability legislation, 21
discrimination, 7, 8, 10
    eliminating, 48
    forms of, 85
    government and, 21
    local needs targeting and, 52–53, 126
    in medical journals, 54
    mental health literacy, prejudice
        and, 79, 80f
    mental illness and, 16–17, 32
documentation, 49

ECT. See electroconvulsive therapy
education, 42
    biomedically oriented model of, 65
    contact-based, 115–16f, 121, 122, 131
    medical, 60
    prejudice and, 67–69
    stereotypes and, 117
    videos for, 116–18
Egypt, 34
electroconvulsive therapy (ECT), 15, 106
embarrassment, 40
emergency departments, 114–15
employment, 10t
    disabilities and, 22–24
    inequity, 22–24
    mental health and, 21
empowerment, 94, 144
enlightened opportunism, 41–44, 49, 68, 127
environments, stigma and, 84–85
etiological theories, 4, 34, 86, 110
eugenics movement, 4
European Union, 104
    deinstitutionalization in, 89
    Green Paper, 91
    state psychiatric beds in, 90t
evaluation, 81–84, 132, 162, 169
    anonymity/confidentiality, 178–79
    of behavior, 173f
    black box, 170
    challenges of, 177–78
    communicating results of, 180
    comparison groups and, 179
    cycle, 171f

evaluation (*Cont.*)
    data collection plan, 175–76, 177*f*
    data management and analysis, 175–76
    design, 179
    erroneous results in, 178
    ethical issues in, 178–80
    ethics clearance in, 179–80
    identification of lessons learned in, 176–78
    one group, pre-test post-test design, 171
    performance targets of, 174–75
    of personal stigma, 173*f*
    of social distance, 174*f*
evidence-based advocacy. *See* scientific
    evidence
evidence-based medicine, 70

family
    anti-stigma programs and, 164–65
    honor, 35–36
    stigma consequences for, 6, 10*t*, 11–12
fighting stigma, 112–13
finances, 140–43
focus groups, 145–50
    checklist, 149*f*
    conducting, 145–47
    consent form, 148*f*
    data, analysis of, 149–50
    discussions, 148–49
    troubleshooting, 147–49
folk psychiatry, 76–77
forensic mental health systems, 92
freedom, 103
Freud, Sigmund, 111
Friern Hospital, 86
funding, 71
funding application, 141–42

General Social Survey, 108
Global Burden of Disease Study, 12
goals, anti-stigma program, 48–49, 129*t*–130*t*,
    138–39*f*, 162–63
Goffman, Erving, 5, 88
government, discrimination and, 21
grassroots initiatives, 43–44, 46
Greece, 112
group learning, 45

health-care systems
    Chinese, 31
    stigma in general, 60–61, 93–94

health professionals, 158
homelessness, 27–28
honor, 35–36
hospitalization, involuntary, 109*f*
hospitals. *See also* asylums
    budgets, 87
    emergency departments in, 114–15
    Islamic, 33, 35
    Public perception of, 88–91
    U.S. state, 87–88
housing, 10*t*, 27, 113–14
hsiao, 35
human rights. *See* rights
Hungary, 89

identity
    diagnosis and, 58, 64
    mental illness and, 5, 58
    spoiled, 5
ierkegaard, Soren, 3
Indian culture, stigma in, 38–40
INDIGO. *See* International Study of
    Discrimination and Stigma Outcomes
individualism, 34
information campaigns, 73. *See also*
    social-marketing campaigns
Institute of Psychiatry, 18
institutionalization, 86–91, 87*f*, 88–89, 90*t*, 91
institutional racism, 84–85
insurance, 32
interest, creating, 139–40
International Pilot Study of Schizophrenia
    (IPSS), 31
International Study of Discrimination and
    Stigma Outcomes (INDIGO), 10
intervention
    cognitive-therapy, 74
    community-level, 42–43
    defining success of, 81–84
inverse law care, 27–28
involuntary treatment, 20
IPSS. *See* International Pilot Study of
    Schizophrenia
Islamic culture, stigma in, 33–35
Italy, 89

Japan, 36, 37
jinn, 34
Jofré, Gilbert, 4
journalists, 121, 156–57, 165

Kennedy, John F., 89
King's College, 18
knowledge
    anti-stigma programs and medical, 76–77
    attitude-behavior continuum, 78–79f
    of mental illness in China, 37t
    prejudice and, 70–73
Koran, 34

labeling, 3, 5, 5n1. *See also* diagnosis
    attribution theory and, 6–7
    careless use of, 64
    fear of, 9
    stereotypes and, 6–7
"Labeling Theory," 88
leadership, 45–47, 127
lead organization governance, 45
legislation
    civil-commitment, 61–62
    disability, 21
legislators, 160
Like Minds, Like Mine, 16–17, 82
literacy-based programs, 73
literacy theory, 73
living factor, 36
Local Action Groups, 44
local needs, 52–53, 126
logic model. *See* program logic model
Long Island, 25–26
low-cost housing, 27

madness, 35, 37
magnuun, 35
majnoon, 34
Malleus Maleficarum, 3–4
maltreatment, 33–34
mandated care, 58, 62–63
mark of shame, 3
marriage, 36, 40
Maslow, Abraham, 96
McLuhan, Marshal, 84
media. *See also* social-marketing campaigns
    advertising, 18, 166
    anti-stigma programs targeting,
        120–22
    arts, 166
    campaigns, 96–98
    CNN effect, 99
    experts, external, 166
    mental health journalism, 121

mental illness depiction in, 28–30, 100,
        120–22
    news, 29
    radio campaigns, 97, 98f, 99, 166
    reliance on, 96–98
    schizophrenia and, 120–21
    stereotypes in, 17
    television, 166
    usage in anti-stigma programs,
        165–66
medical education, 60
medicalizing, 76, 77
medical journals, stigma in, 53, 54f
medical knowledge, 76–77
medication, 6, 58
    cost of, 65
    negativity toward, 106
    side-effects of, 64–65
medicine, evidence-based, 70
Medline, 54
mental abnormality, mental illness and, 76–77
mental health, 13–14
    abuse and, 32, 87
    budget, 14
    Canadian understanding of, 71–72
    country income and, 14t
    employment and, 21
    funding, 71
    Indian conception of, 39
    inverse law care, 27–28
    journalism, 121
    legal aspects of, 20–21
    NIMBY and, 24–26, 113–14
    policy, 86, 104, 160
    poverty and, 21
    reform, 91
    services, 27–28
mental health care providers, 58
The Mental Health Commission of Canada,
        121
    Opening Minds, 10, 18–19, 123, 141,
        173f–174f
mental health development, 20–22
Mental Health First Aid, 74–76
mental health literacy, 71–72, 74–76
    definition of, 73
    information campaigns for, 73
    Mental Health First Aid, 74–76
    of police, 159
    population-based campaign for, 73–74

mental health literacy (*Cont.*)
  prejudice and discrimination, 79, 80*f*
  social-marketing campaigns, 101
  stigma and, 74, 76
  theory, 73
mental health professionals, 158
  anti-stigma programs and, 57–59
  attitudes of, 63–64
  credibility of, 127
  pessimism of, 59
  police power of, 104
  public image of, 106
  solutions for, 63–66
  stereotypes held by, 59
  stigma of, 114, 127
  terminology of, 64
mental health programs, 58
mental health systems, 20
  forensic, 92
  recovery-oriented, 94–95
  as social control, 61–63
  stigma consequences and, 12–16, 57
mental illness. *See also* labeling;
    stereotypes
  behavior and, 69–70
  beliefs about, 34, 35, 39
  Canadian attitude toward, 88
  cause of, 39, 42, 72
  in China, knowledge of, 37*t*
  concealment of, 11
  conception of, 76
  consequences of, 42
  contact-based education for patients with,
    115, 116*f*
  criminality and, 28
  definition of, 69, 77
  delivery of anti-stigma programs and
    experience of, 163–64
  demystification of, 71
  diagnostic overshadowing of, 60, 93
  disability and, 12–13
  discrimination and, 16–17, 32
  false understanding of, 76
  fear of, 11
  hereditary factors of, 4, 36, 111
  identity and, 5, 58
  insurance and, 32
  in Koran, 34
  media depiction of, 28–30, 100, 120–22
  mental abnormality and, 76–77

  neurobiological factors of, 72–73, 77,
    109–11
  other illness and, 103, 109–11, 128
  police engagement and, 118–20
  prisoners and, 92
  public stigma, 8, 72, 88–91, 108–9, 128
  public tolerance of, 28–30
  re-institutionalization and, 101–2
  relationships and, 29–30
  salary and, 23
  serious, 23, 39, 75, 125
  shame and, 35–37, 40
  sin and, 3, 4
  social relations and, 34–35
  symptoms of, 73, 76, 110, 159, 164
  video education about, 116–18
  violence and, 28, 72, 75, 108–9
monitoring, 51–52, 140–43, 169–70. *See also*
    evaluation
moralizing, 76
movies, 121–22
mutual aid, 41

The National Alliance for the Mentally Ill, 9,
    110
negative stereotypes. *See* stereotypes
neighborhood programs, 113–14, 159
networks
  advantages of, 44–45
  construction of, 45–46
  definition of, 44
  governance and leadership of, 45–47
  of practice, 44–45, 127
  unifying vision of, 46
neurobiological factors, 72–73, 77, 109–11
news media, 29
New Zealand, 16–17
niksala, 38
NIMBY. *See* Not In My Backyard
normality, behavior and, 68–69
Not In My Backyard (NIMBY), 24–25
  in Long Island, 25–26
  overcoming NIMBYism, 113–14
nurses, 60–61

One Flew Over the Cuckoo's Nest, 15, 88
one group, pre-test post-test design, 171
Opening Minds (Mental Health Commission
    of Canada), 10, 18–19, 123, 141,
    173*f*–174*f*

Open–the Doors Global Program to Fight Stigma Because of Schizophrenia (World Psychiatric Association), v, 16, 42, 44, 52, 97, 112, 115, 118
    movies, 121–22
    training manual, 133
OVID, 53–54

pagal, 39
paternalism, 58, 103
pathologizing, 76
patients
    accreditation guidelines for, 116*f*
    rights of, 88, 115
peer-support mental health programs, 58
performance standards, anti-stigma programs, 82
personality disorder, 61, 92
personal stigma, 5–6
pilot-testing, 167*f*, 176
police
    mental health literacy of, 159
    stigma and, 118–20
    target groups, 159–60
    violence and, 119
policy, 41
    makers, 54, 160
    mental health, 86, 104, 160
    scientific evidence-based, 50, 54–55, 180
population-based literacy campaign, 73–74
positional leaders, 46
poverty, 21
practice
    for anti-stigma programs, building better, 49, 53–56
    networks, 44–45, 127
    scientific evidence and, 54, 132
prayer, 34
prejudice
    anti-stigma programs and, 67–69
    definition of, 67
    education and, 67–69
    knowledge and, 70–73
    mental health literacy, discrimination and, 79, 80*f*
    misconception and, 67
    reduction, 79–81
    re-fencing, 71
    theories about, 80
presenteeism, 24

Pressure Point, 88
prisoners, 92
productivity, 24
    presenteeism and, 24
prognosis, 61, 93
program committee, 135, 136*f*, 137
program logic model
    activities, 161, 162*f*
    exit clause of, 163
    objectives of, 162*f*, 163
    resources, 162*f*
psychiatrists. *See* mental health professionals
psychiatry, 14. *See also* anti-psychiatry movement
    community, 91
    folk, 76–77
    nineteenth century, 4
    stigmatization of, 15
    television and, 28
    as weapon, 107
PsychInfo, 54*f*
psychologizing, 77
public
    hospital perception of, 88–91
    meetings, 159
    perception of treatment, 88–91
    relations, 165
    service announcements, 97
    speaking, 164
    stigma, 8, 72, 83, 88–91, 108–9, 128
    tolerance, 28–30
punishment, 34, 35, 39

qualitative data, 170
qualitative investigation, 144–50
quality of life, 125
quarantine, 103
Queen's University, 75

racism, institutional, 84–85
radio campaigns, 97, 98*f*, 99, 166
recovery, 32. *See also* treatment
    active rehabilitation, 95
    in China, philosophy of, 37*t*
    from depression, 59
    oriented mental health systems, 94–95
    paternalism and, 58
    from schizophrenia, 59
    stigma and, 9, 63, 87*f*, 94–95
re-institutionalization, 101–2

relationships, 29–30
religion, 125
reputational leaders, 46
resources, 140–43
rights, 7, 13, 17, 20
    civil, 21, 30
    human, 73, 94, 104, 107
    of patients, 88, 115
    stigma and, 9
risk-management tools, 62
romantic life, 10*t*
Royal College of Psychiatrists, 63
Royal Commission on Psychiatric Services, 88

salary, 23
SAMHSA. *See* Substance Abuse and Mental
    Health Administration
Scheff, Thomas J., 88
schizophrenia, 4, 8, 10, 16, 22, 25, 71
    beliefs about, 34, 38
    cause of, 38
    consequences of, 40
    in developing countries, 31–33
    homelessness and, 27
    IPSS, 31
    long-term outcomes of, 59
    media and, 120–21
    in movies, 121–22
    radio advertisements about, 97,
        98*f*, 99
    recovery from, 59
    social distance and, 29*f*
    violence and, 98–99
Schizophrenia Fellowship of Victoria, 65
Schizophrenia Society of Canada,
    116–17
school, 10*t*
schools, 157–58
scientific evidence, 126
    advocacy through, 50–51, 55
    defining, 51
    monitoring, 51–52
    perception of, 51–52
    policy and, 50, 54–55, 180
    practice and, 54, 132
    situational analysis and, 53
scientific presentations, 180
Scientology. *See* Church of Scientology
See Me (Scotland), 17, 78–79, 83–84
sekela, 38

self-acceptance, 94
self-esteem, 8, 9, 65
self-harm, 61
self-help, 41, 107
self-help treatment, 73
self-mortification, 88
self-reflection, 176
self-stigma, 8, 32–33, 77, 138
semi-structured interviews, 150
    before and after, 152
    administration of, 153
    cost of, 152
    demographic of, 153
    designing, 152–53
    instruments of, 153
    letter to participants of, 154*f*
    objectives of, 152
    questions, 151*f*
    readability of, 152–53
    tracking participants, 153
serious mental illness, 23, 39, 75, 125
shame, 35–37, 40
shared governance, 45
ships of fools, 104
shock therapy. *See* electroconvulsive therapy
side-effects (medication), 64–65
sin, 3, 4
situational analysis, 53
slaves, 3
The Snake Pit, 88
soap operas, 120
social control, mental health systems as, 61–63
social distance, 60, 75, 110, 123, 128
    in China, 36, 37*t*, 38
    evaluation of, 174*f*
    schizophrenia and, 29*f*
    social-marketing campaign and, 98
social exclusion, 57
social inclusion, 95, 131
    social-marketing campaigns and, 99–102
socialization, 84
social-marketing campaigns, 96, 128.
        See also media
    anti-stigma programs, 70–71, 100*t*
    of Church of Scientology, 107–8
    culture and, 102
    mental health literacy, 101
    principles of, 101
    on radio, 97, 98*f*, 99, 166
    social distance and, 98

social inclusion and, 99–102
  targeting, 101
social oppression, 7, 21, 84
social relations, 34–35
social structures, 85
social tolerance, 77
society
  culture and, 102
  stigma consequences and, 12–16
speaker programs, 164
spoiled identity, 5
stereotypes, 3–4, 5, 36, 41, 91
  dangerousness, 100
  doctors/nurses, 93
  education and, 117
  labeling and, 6–7
  media and, 17
  mental health care professionals and, 59
  nurses beliefs and, 60–61
  public stigma, 8, 72, 83, 88–91, 108–9, 128
  self-stigma and, 8
  violence as, 61–62, 72
stigma, v, 5, 16. *See also* anti-stigma programs;
    courtesy stigma
  in Balinese culture, 38
  beliefs about, 112
  in Chinese culture, 35–36, 37*t*, 38
  community care and, 87*f*, 91–94
  consequences of, 5, 8–9, 10*t*, 139–40
  definition of, 3, 7, 18
  in developing countries, 31–33
  emergency departments and, 114–15
  environments and, 84–85
  evaluation of personal, 173*f*
  family consequences and, 6, 10*t*, 11–12
  fear of, 34
  fighting, 112–13
  in general health-care systems, 60–61,
    93–94
  growing interest in, 51
  in Indian culture, 38–40
  institutionalization and, 86–91, 87*f*, 88–89,
    90*t*, 91
  in Islamic culture, 33–35
  literature, 83, 161
  in medical journals, 53, 54*f*
  from mental health care providers, 58
  mental health literacy and, 74, 76
  of mental health professionals, 114, 127
  mental health systems, societies, and

consequences of, 12–16, 57
  nature of, 129*t*
  origins and meaning of, 3–7, 129*t*
  in other cultures, 33–40, 125–26
  personal, 5–6
  police and, 118–20
  public, 8, 72, 83, 88–91, 108–9, 128
  recovery and, 9, 63, 87*f*, 94–95
  reduction, 40, 66
  rights and, 9
  self, 8, 32–33, 138
Stigma: Notes on the Management of Spoiled
    Identity (Goffman), 5, 88
stigma-by-association, 11
  wise normals, 11n2
stigmata, 3
stigmatization
  definition of, 7
  medicalizing, 77
  moralizing, 76
  pathologizing, 76
  of psychiatry, 15
  psychologizing, 77
  social oppression and, 84
  vicious cycles of, 6
Substance Abuse and Mental Health
    Administration (SAMHSA), 17–18
suicide, 23, 35–36, 61
surveys. *See* semi-structured interviews

target groups
  health professionals, 158
  journalists, 156–57
  members of community neighborhoods,
    113–14, 159
  mental health professionals, 158
  police, 159–60
  policy makers/legislators, 160
  schools, 157–58
  youth, 157–58
targeting, 48, 127–28, 129*t*, 131
  local needs, 52–53, 126
  media, 120–22
  social-marketing campaigns, 101
television, 120
  for children, 28–29
  using, 166
Telling Is Risky Business, 9
Time to Change, 18
Together Against Stigma, 112

Tooting Bec Hospital, 113–14
transinstitutionalization, 91–92
treatment. *See also* coercive treatment;
    recovery
  in Australia, 93
  availability of, 73
  community care, 92–93
  of depression, 73
  equitable, 65
  forced confinement and, 103–4, 105*f*, 111
  gap, 92
  in India, 39
  orders, community, 104
  overshadowing, 60
  public perception of, 88–91
  quality of, 93–94
  self-harm, 61
  self-help, 73
  trust, 63

unemployment, 22
United Nations, 113
United Nations Convention on the Rights of
    Persons with Disabilities, 7, 13, 84
United Nations Declaration on the Rights of
    People with Disability, 21
unpredictability, violence and, 108–9
UN Resolution 46-119, 13

vicious cycles of stigmatization, 6
videos, educational, 116–18

violence
  mental illness and, 28, 72, 75, 108–9
  police and, 119
  schizophrenia and, 98–99
  as stereotype, 61–62, 72
  unpredictability and, 108–9
volunteers, 55

weakness, 38
What a Difference a Friend Makes, 18
White Noise, 121
WHO. *See* World Health Organization
wise normals, 11n2
witches, 3–4
The Witches' Hammer, 3–4
work. *See* employment
World Association of Social Psychiatry, 112
The World Disability Report, 12
World Health Day, 112
World Health Organization (WHO), 20, 31,
    112
  Mental Health Atlas Project, 13, 14*f*, 89–90
World Psychiatric Association, v, 15, 16,
    18–19, 42, 63, 97
  General Assembly, 112–13
  Task Force on the Destigmatization of
    Psychiatry and Psychiatrists, 106

youth, 157–58

zoning laws, 24–26